615.321
N234d

AGK1419-1

CH

DISCOVER
ESSENTIAL OILS

DISCOVER
ESSENTIAL OILS

NICOLA NAYLOR

Ulysses Press ⚒ Berkeley, CA
1998

Published by: Ulysses Press
    P.O. Box 3440
    Berkeley, CA 94703-3440

Library of Congress Catalog Card Number: 97-61009

ISBN: 1-56975-080-7

Printed in Canada by Best Book Manufacturers

First published as *Healing with Essential Oils*, Gill & Macmillan, 1996

10 9 8 7 6 5 4 3 2 1

Editorial and production: Lily Chou
Typesetter: David Wells
Cover Design: B & L Design
Indexer: Sayre Van Young

Distributed in the United States by Publishers Group West and in Canada by Raincoast Books

ACKNOWLEDGEMENTS

I would like to thank my editor, Tessa Strickland, for all her help and encouragement, and my copy editor, Kate Parker, for being so meticulous. Thank you, also, to all my clients, to whom I am indebted—it is only through experience that one can truly learn anything. A special thanks to the former Inner London Education Authority and in particular to Battersea and Clapham Education Institute, without whom I would never have embarked on this profession.

TABLE OF CONTENTS

Chapter One
What Are Essential Oils? 1

Chapter Two
The History of Healing with Essential Oils 7

Chapter Three
Helping Yourself to Health with Essential Oils 12

Chapter Four
Safety with Essential Oils 16

Chapter Five
Chemistry and Botany 22

Chapter Six
Healing at Home 34

Chapter Seven
Healing Methods 46

Chapter Eight
Using Vegetable and Macerated Oils 63

Chapter Nine
Buying and Storing Essential Oils 72

Chapter Ten
Essential Oils in Health Care Settings 79

Chapter Eleven
Professional Treatment with Essential Oils 83

Chapter Twelve
Case Studies 88

Helpful Addresses 100

Recommended Reading 105

Index 107

WHAT ARE
ESSENTIAL OILS?

"The way to health is to have an aromatic bath and scented massage every day." This was the advice given by the Greek doctor Hippocrates, the father of Western medicine. I, for one, cannot think of a more pleasurable way of keeping well. People of the ancient world knew about the relaxing and protective powers of plant oils; they used them to guard themselves against contagious diseases and infections.

The therapeutic aims and methods of using aromatics have not changed fundamentally since the times of Hippocrates, but they have expanded and improved. With today's scientific knowledge we understand more about why essential oils have either antiviral, antifungal or antibacterial properties. The fact that I have been in regular daily contact with essential oils through my work as an aromatologist over the last ten years and have never had so much as a cold speaks for their protective and health-giving properties.

THE SOURCES OF ESSENTIAL OILS

The pure, fragrant substances extracted from aromatic plants are known as *essential oils*. This does not mean that these oils are essential to the life of the plants from which they originate. Rather, the term is used to suggest that the oils contain the healing *essence* of the plants. Unlike the vegetable and macerated oils in which they can be diluted, essential oils are volatile and non-greasy.

Essential oils are contained in the glands, sacs, veins and glandular hairs concentrated in different parts of the plant. For instance, myrtle oil is extracted from the young leaves and twigs of the small myrtle tree. Marjoram comes from the flowering tops of the herb, while spruce comes from the needles of the spruce tree. Ylang ylang is extracted from flowers and cinnamon from leaves or bark. Citrus oils such as orange, lime and lemon are squeezed from the peel of the fruit, while vetiver is extracted from the root, ginger from the rhizome and black pepper from the seeds.

METHODS OF APPLICATION

I work with around one hundred oils that I dilute in vegetable oil and apply in massage treatments. I also bottle oils for home use by my clients. Sometimes I use just one essential oil; at other times I combine two or more oils. My practice is busy with people seeking help for a wide range of health complaints. I select the oils and the best way to apply them according to the individual client's needs. Oil massage is the usual form of treatment because the essential oil is quickly absorbed through the skin and carried by the blood around the body. After six to ten hours it is eliminated from the body (leaving no toxic residue, as far as tests have shown) through the urine, feces, perspiration or simply exhalation.

Professional aromatologists may also give essential oils as intramuscular injections or internally, mixed with honey water or made into a tablet. Do not use these methods yourself unless you have had professional training. However, there are many ways in which you can use essential oils therapeutically at home: in baths — including sitz, hand and foot baths — compresses, inhalations, ointments, lotions and creams as well as in massage treatment. (See Chapter Seven for details of these methods.)

Methods of Extraction

Steam distillation has been the most widely practiced way of extracting the oils from the plants since the time of Avicenna (980–1037 A.D.), a Persian physician who revolutionized the rudimentary methods of distillation. The advantage of steam distillation is that it lets through only the tiniest molecules, those which make up an essential oil. The larger molecules, including those forming pesticides, fertilizers or other non-volatile chemical compounds, are left behind and therefore do not contaminate the pure essential oil.

The best citrus essential oil is obtained by *cold pressing* or *expression* since steam distillation does not produce oil with the same composition as that present in the fruit itself. During cold pressing the oil is squeezed out from the oil glands under the surface of the rind. Because the larger molecules from chemical fruit sprays penetrate these glands, they find their way into the extracted oil, so it is important to use untreated crops.

Carbon dioxide extraction and *percolation* are two methods that have been developed relatively recently and, like cold pressing, yield a product that closely resembles the oil as it is contained in the plant. The carbon method involves the use of very expensive equipment while the percolation process seems to be more economical, with promising results.

Solvent extraction produces substances known as absolutes and resinoids, which are, strictly speaking, not considered to be essential oils but rather the concentrated material from which perfume is made. Jasmine absolute, sandalwood or frankincense resin will contain all the plant molecules soluble in the hydrocarbon or alcohol solvent used in the extraction process. Some of the solvent will also remain in the end product, however. Sensitivity to these solvents is not uncommon and is certainly undesirable.

Solvent extraction is the most ancient method of obtaining aromatic substances. We owe a lot of what we know about essential oils to the methods used to obtain the sweet-smelling pomades that our ancestors wore in order to ward off disease and insects, or the embalming resins used by the Egyptians for their ability to preserve. But these aromatic compounds are no longer considered suitable for therapeutic use today.

This does not mean that I have not frequently enjoyed giving and receiving a massage or bath scented with jasmine or tuberose absolute. The smell is divine and has a positive psychological effect, just as a synthetic smell can have, but there is little medicinal value in such absolutes compared with that of true essential oils. Absolutes offer an aromatic, uplifting experience, not a way of healing.

THE MARKETING OF ESSENTIAL OILS

As a practitioner, I want the natural, unadulterated oil — nothing added or taken away. This is not easy to come by because many growers and dealers have not heard of using essential oils for health care. They are used to altering the natural balance of chemical components within the oil to produce a standardized product for the perfume or food industry. Since these are still the biggest markets for essential oils, their requirements control the production.

I have traveled extensively in India to research the use of massage and essential oils in ayurvedic practice — Indian herbal medicine. During my travels I met countless representatives from the perfume and the food and flavorings industries who all insisted that their standardized products were essential oils. They even offered to tailor make them for me!

Sometimes I found the oils were tampered with in the interest of shady commercialism. It is possible to take the cheap and easily available ingredient of one oil and add it to another. The claim of having a pure essential oil can still be made. An added compound can be detected only by an experienced "nose."

ANALYZING ESSENTIAL OILS

Each essential oil contains a hundred or more natural chemical compounds. The composition of an oil relates directly to its beneficial effects or hazards. This knowledge enables us to choose the oil most likely to help with a particular condition.

Variations in species, as well as changes in growing and climatic conditions, can alter the composition of an oil. The chemical make-up is also different in different plants and varies between species and even hybrids of the same species.

The usual way of determining the chemical components of an oil is by using a device known as a *gas-liquid chromatograph*. Using this device most good oil suppliers will take a reading for each batch of oil — information that, along with the date of production, is not commonly available to purchasers. However, some reputable suppliers with mail-order lists will give these details on request. (A selection of these can be found at the back of the book under "Aromatherapy Products" in the "Helpful Addresses" section.)

BUYING ESSENTIAL OILS

If you choose to buy essential oils from a store, it is best to go to a specialist in natural health products, such as a health food store, and not somewhere selling perfumed cosmetics or toiletries. Look for pure essential oils, not blends that are ready mixed in a vegetable "carrier" oil. You should buy oils in dark-glass bottles with screw tops and droppers for dispensing. They should be kept for no longer than two years and stored in a cool, dark place out of the reach of children. (See Chapter Nine.)

Ten oils are sufficient for basic and first-aid healing at home (see Chapter Six). There is also a wide variety of additional oils that you can add to your collection, although their therapeutic uses are less well established from a scientific perspective. These include oils such as patchouli (*Pogostemon patchouli*) and vetiver (*Vetiveria zizanioides*). There are several varieties of plants, such as basil and thyme, all of which yield oils with varying properties. This makes them complex for home use. Since it is still difficult to identify oils of a particular species of, for instance, lavender or eucalyptus from the store, and nearly impossible to know the exact proportions of the chemicals contained in the bottle you buy, I will give a general guide to the contents of the most commonly available essential oils and their therapeutic methods and uses.

A properly qualified aromatologist should be consulted for the treatment of more serious health complaints. (See the "Helpful Addresses" section at the back of this book.)

2

THE HISTORY OF HEALING WITH ESSENTIAL OILS

The history of healing with essential oils has often been confused with the history of perfumery or of herbalism. Perfumery is the non-medicinal use of aromatic substances while herbalism is the medicinal use of the whole plant.

Herbalism and perfumery have their roots buried deep in the rituals and customs of ancient civilizations, while aromatherapy, which uses distilled or expressed essential oils therapeutically, is a comparatively recent development. Indeed, essential oils only became available in quantity following advances in distillation methods. The term *aromatherapy* was coined in the early twentieth century. Over the last few years the word *aromatology* has emerged to further emphasize the medicinal and clinical use of the pure aromatic part of the plant: the essential oil. Otherwise the two terms can, to a large extent, be used interchangeably.

ANCIENT TIMES

It is often difficult to know whether references in ancient scriptures to the use of aromatic plants like sandalwood, ginger, myrrh and calamus indicate the essential oil or the plant in its entirety. Even when we find mention of aromatic substances, these would often have been extracted by the use of fats and waxes — as illustrated in the Egyptian paintings of jars filled with aromatic unguents — and would therefore not have been pure.

Herbalism was certainly widespread in Indian, Egyptian, Greek and Roman societies. We can read their works of reference such as *De materia medica* by the first-century Roman physician Dioscorides and *The Book of Healing* by the tenth-century Persian Avicenna, referred to in the previous chapter. These texts record the healing properties of plants, not necessarily those of individual essential oils.

Before Avicenna — to whom, as we have seen, we also owe the most significant advance in steam distillation — rudimentary forms of distillation did exist, but it was mainly used in order to extract exotic flower waters. The essential oil produced was an almost negligible by-product, as flowers like rose and neroli contain only minute amounts of oil.

THE MIDDLE AGES TO THE EIGHTEENTH CENTURY

Throughout the Middle Ages and on into the seventeenth and eighteenth centuries, the healing power of herbs was recognized and herbalism was practiced. Across Europe aromatic plants were cultivated in the gardens of monasteries and stately homes; in the fourteenth century knowledge of the curative properties of herbs was prevalent among the rural population during the bubonic plague, or Black Death, when herbs were noted for their antiseptic effect. By 1535, Grasse, in southern France, was established as a center for making perfumes using chemical compounds and essential oils. Perfumes were not just valued as a way of masking unpleasant smells but also for their protective powers against disease.

However, the first recorded recognition of the healing potential of distilled essential oils, as opposed to herbs and plants in general, was made by the Swiss physician and alchemist Paracelsus (1493–1541). In his work *The Great Surgery Book* he noted that the task of alchemy was not to make gold from base metals but to develop medicines from plants. He saw distillation as the way to produce the *quinta essentia*, the "healing essence" of a plant.

After this we find mention of essential oils in the official pharmacopoeias of the time. Rosemary, cedarwood, juniper, sage and lavender oils were known to seventeenth-century pharmacists and used mostly for their antiseptic qualities.

Paracelsus was also important for the link he established between essential oils and chemistry. Today a basic understanding of the natural chemical properties of essential oils and their actions is the key to successful healing work.

THE TWENTIETH CENTURY

By the twentieth century chemical science was becoming very popular. In the world of medicine, individual plant properties were isolated, or even synthesized, and used as drugs. In aromatherapy we do not separate the individual chemical components of an essential oil, nor do we use a reconstituted oil. Increasingly, we try to research the therapeutic value of the hundred or more chemicals contained in each oil so that we can understand what effect the whole oil may have when used in treatment.

A few scientists, mainly in Europe, began this process earlier this century. The best known was René-Maurice Gattefossé, who coined the word *aromatherapy*. He is also the man renowned for badly burning his arm in his laboratory and for the discovery he made as a result. He is said to have plunged his burned arm in a vat of lavender because it was the only cold liquid he could quickly find. The pain lessened so significantly and the wound healed so quickly with little scarring that he was inspired to find out more about the healing properties of essential oils. Indeed, he and others used essential oils on soldiers wounded in the trenches during World War I.

Since then, aromatherapy has been widely used for medicinal purposes in France, some of the most informative books having been written by French practitioners. Among these are Dr. Jean Valnet's *The Practice of Aromatherapy*; and *Aromathérapie exactement* by Pierre Franchomme, an aromatologist. Dr. Pénoël, a medical doctor, has prescribed essential oils as part of the complementary medicine he practices. I have attended some of Dr. Pénoël's lectures in which he showed slides demonstrating some startling results, even in cases of advanced cancer.

AROMATHERAPY

Aromatherapy was established in Britain in the 1950s through the beauty industry by Australian Marguerite Maury. She was interested in the ability of essential oils to penetrate the skin and preserve youth. Her cosmetic use of essential oils was soon extended into the beauty salons where beauticians were trained to give an aromatherapeutic massage for relaxation and skin care. This type of aromatherapy is now commonly practiced in countries such as Australia, the U.S., Canada and throughout Scandinavia. I prefer to call it an *aromatic massage* to avoid any claim to therapy suggested in the word *aromatherapy*.

Beauticians are not qualified to "treat" any medical condition and they tend to use ready-blended oils. Short courses in aromatherapy rarely equip anyone to mix oils for medicinal use.

AROMATOLOGY

Since the late 1980s a few training schools have begun to teach the basic medical, chemical, physical and botanical science necessary for therapists to work therapeutically with essential oils. Such therapists or *aromatologists*, as well as specially trained nurses and midwives, are now working with essential oils in hospitals, hospices and private practices all over the world (see Chapter Ten).

An aromatologist will use only pure, distilled or expressed essential oils that are based on a scientific understanding, acquired through training, of their properties and effects.

It is important to remember that, before distillation, aromas were extracted mainly by solvents. These are not essential oils but, together with the whole plant, they form the origins of herbalism and perfumery out of which grew aromatherapy. Their history has been summarized here to put the much shorter history of healing with essential oils into historical context, and also because some of the traditional uses of herbs point the way to many of the benefits that have been validated in the therapeutic use of essential oils today.

3

HELPING YOURSELF TO HEALTH WITH ESSENTIAL OILS

THE PLACE FOR COMPLEMENTARY CARE

Modern orthodox medicine has revolutionized the quality and length of human life in the developed countries of the world. Diseases that killed a hundred years ago can now be prevented or cured with vaccinations or drugs. Intricate surgery has saved thousands of lives, while tuberculosis, hepatitis and even pneumonia no longer massacre whole populations the way they once did.

There has been a backlash, however. The drugs themselves have produced some serious side effects that then also need to be treated. Other problems with our modern system of health care include the rising costs of equipment and treatment, hospital bed shortages and the commercial self-interest that promotes research programs that do not always provide cures.

Rather than eradicating ill health, technological advances and affluence have brought new kinds of illness. In place of dysentery and malnutrition we now have obesity, colon cancer and coronary heart disease.

Since our traditional health care system has increasingly failed people over the last twenty years, there has been a rise in the popularity of alternative or complementary medicine. Ten years ago, when I was first starting my practice, almost no one had heard of an aromatherapist. Now, there may be some misconceptions about exactly what I do, but I am not met with the same ignorance or skepticism. Aromatherapy has taken root and spread more in Great Britain than in any other country.

Sadly, people still come to me and other complementary therapists as the last resort after a round of fruitless visits to conventional doctors. In frustration or desperation, they turn to natural medicine either because they have found no cure for their eczema, arthritis or whatever their problems might be, or because they can no longer tolerate the side effects of the drugs they were prescribed to suppress the symptoms of their disease. Even at this late stage they may find a cure or safe form of relief by using natural products like essential oils. And even if the treatment with essential oils is only palliative, at least there is no risk of drug-induced disease or undesirable side effects.

Taking Responsibility for Your Health

Many illnesses and complaints are the result of personal neglect and ignorance. If you can recognize the early signs of conditions such as premenstrual syndrome (PMS), tiredness or sinusitis, and know how to relieve them using natural, non-toxic remedies, you can then manage your health and save yourself from more serious illness. Taking responsibility for your health also means following a diet that is low in sugars, fats, refined foods and alcohol, and high in fresh fruit, vegetables, legumes and grains. Try to strike a balance between exercise and rest, especially if you have a sedentary job.

Doctors frequently prescribe antibiotics for people with colds or flu symptoms who want to keep up with the demands of the office or the family. The danger of antibiotics is that they work indiscriminately, killing both the beneficial as well as the unfriendly bacteria, thus upsetting the delicate balance of intestinal flora. Ultimately, digestive problems or vaginal thrush can result. Antibiotics should be reserved for saving lives, for which they deserve full credit, and not used to treat minor illnesses, since they can do as much harm as good.

A QUICK FIX

We are a drug-dependent culture, whether it be for stimulants like caffeine, alcohol, cigarettes or chocolate, or for the "quick-fix" nature of painkillers and tranquilizers. We ignore the long-term consequences of our addictions in favor of short-term relief. The more we take drugs, the less effective they become. Our bodies grow to resist them and at the same time we feel we need more and more.

Alternative therapists often view pain, high blood pressure or fever as an indicator of underlying problems that need to be dealt with by natural remedies, not masked with painkillers, blood thinners, inhalants, antihistamines, antidepressants, diuretics or a cocktail of these. It is worth trying a massage with essential oils to relieve stress and tension before reaching for the sedatives. If you suffer from asthma, try an oil inhalation before continually sniffing Ventolin.

Faced with someone having a heart attack or injured in an accident, I would be among the first to call for an ambulance. There are all sorts of conditions, from broken bones to aneurysms to the acute pain suffered in some terminal illnesses, which need the skills and attention that only traditional medical care offers. However, there are many conditions that can be treated naturally and benignly. Essential oils are not a guaranteed cure-all but should be the first port of call before taking such drugs as steroids or even aspirin.

The professionalization of health care, with the use of high-tech equipment and scientific terminology, has played a part in creating the passive patient. The miraculous power of drugs to cure once incurable diseases became personified in the doctor. The idea that the doctor could chase away all complaints and the patient need do nothing for himself had not been challenged until recently. Now there is a growing awareness of the limitations of conventional medical practice.

Natural Self-Help

This is not to suggest that we should play doctors and nurses; merely that through lifestyle management we can try to prevent ill health. Through the use of natural products we can safely take charge of applying first aid and can cope with common, minor ailments.

By describing a basic selection of essential oils and their uses, I hope to empower those interested in taking responsibility for their own health at a daily functional level. For more complicated conditions, I advise a consultation with a conventional doctor, an aromatologist or any qualified complementary practitioner of your choice.

4

SAFETY WITH ESSENTIAL OILS

Essential oils can be harmful when misused, overused or otherwise abused. Like other household products such as bleach, alcohol or matches, they are hazardous if not stored and used with care.

Most substances are dangerous when used in excess and essential oils are no different, especially when they are taken internally. For example, I know about the harm done by an essential oil in an accidental overdose. A four-year-old child swallowed 5 to 8 ml of clove oil (*Syzygium aromaticum*), after which her nervous system was compromised and she lost consciousness. After a worrisome twenty-four hours in intensive care she recovered and later regained full health. The same precautions, such as keeping bottles out of the reach of children, should apply to essential oils as it does to any other medicines.

SOME SAFETY TIPS

Essential oils are highly concentrated and powerful products. Some basic but important safety measures to remember are:

- keep essential oils out of the reach of children

- buy and store undiluted essential oils in bottles with integral drop dispensers to minimize the risk of overdosing (only one drop at a time will be released)

- never take essential oils internally unless under the advice of a trained practitioner

- never apply essential oils directly to the skin, except in special circumstances for lavender (*Lavandula angustifolia*) or tea tree (*Melaleuca alternifolia*)

- never store essential oils near a heat source or allow them to come into contact with an exposed flame because they are highly flammable

- never allow essential oils to come into contact with the eyes; if they do, wash out the eyes and seek medical help if stinging persists

- do not massage the essential oils into any area of the body where there is an infection, inflammation, varicose veins or recent scarring or fracture; do not massage in cases of fever or high temperature — compresses or other methods of application may be suitable.

SAFE QUANTITIES AND METHODS OF USE

Taking essential oils internally should only be done under the professional supervision of an aromatologist. Ingestion allows the complete and immediate entry of the oil into the body, whereas the amount of oil that can be introduced through the skin or by inhalation is far smaller. By following the methods of application recommended in this book and by mixing the advised, minimal proportions of 1 to 3 percent — around 50 drops in 100 ml of carrier oil — or 6 to 8 drops in a bath, you will be operating within tried and tested safe limits.

MISINFORMATION

Books and media reports on essential oils published in recent years have dispensed rules and advice on "hazardous oils," "oils never to be used in pregnancy" and so on. Unnecessary alarm is caused by quoting research data taken out of the context about the small quantities and external methods of application generally used in aromatology. The reports often fail to specify whether the cited dangers are a result of internal or external usage; they rarely define which species of plant the "culprit" oil comes from and seldom stipulate the quantity of oil necessary to cause observable ill effects. In addition many studies have been based on animal testing, which cannot provide conclusive evidence for human responses.

THE DIFFERENT EFFECTS OF USING HERBAL REMEDIES OR ESSENTIAL OILS

Uncertainty in this area is due to a genuine lack of knowledge about the physiological effects, both good and bad, essential oils can have. Much of our understanding about the therapeutic possibilities of essential oils has been extrapolated from findings about the medicinal properties of entire herbs. There has, therefore, been a tendency to attribute to essential oils the indications and the contraindications listed for herbs.

This is easily done since there is indeed some overlap in the benefits derived from the whole-plant extracts and its aromatics. I can remember strolling in the gardens of several research centers in India discussing the medicinal applications of many of the plants used in Indian herbalism. I found myself equating these with the therapeutics of essential oils. It was tempting to marvel over the general, but often superficial, similarities and to overlook the differences.

Herbal extracts do differ chemically from essential oils. They consist of larger molecules and other chemical structures that are excluded in distillation. They may or may not contain the aromatic molecules of which the distilled essential oils are exclusively composed. These variables lead to differences in both the benefits and the undesirable effects of using either therapeutically.

In the world of perfumery and herbalism there are many plants noted for their toxicity, most of which do not yield an essential oil. Those that do, like pennyroyal (*Mentha pulegium*), are not commonly available, thereby avoiding any doubt or confusion about toxicity. The ten essential oils described in Chapter Six are the most frequently used and well known.

A WORD OF CAUTION

All this is not to say that essential oils do not have the potential to do harm. Insufficient research has been conducted on essential oils and their effects on people. Although we are beginning to recognize both the health giving and the more problematic properties of individual chemical groups in an essential oil, we still do not know how these change when all the groups within the oil interact.

However, it is important to make use of what knowledge we do have about the components of essential oils and their effects. Problems are most likely to arise with those oils containing the chemical compounds known as ketones, phenols, aldehydes or furocoumarins (see Chapter Five). These substances may act as sensitizers, or cause a sensitivity to the sun, or irritate the skin of some people when oils are mixed and applied incorrectly.

CORRECT IDENTIFICATION

All oils should be sold with labels that state the plant and species from which they are distilled as well as the major chemical components. Oils that are considered to be particularly powerful because of the chemical components present, such as sage (*Salvia officinalis*), hyssop (*Hyssopus officinalis*) and some varieties of thyme (e.g. *Thymus vulgaris* ct thujanol-4), should only be bought by trained professionals who can make good use of them within safe limits.

ALLERGIC REACTIONS, INTOLERANCE AND SENSITIZATION

It is believed that allergies — which trigger, for example, asthma, eczema and migraines — are due to an enzyme deficiency in the digestive system. If the enzyme responsible for breaking down a particular protein is missing, the protein molecule will enter the bloodstream unmodified and be treated as a foreign body. The allergic reaction is more acute but similar to an intolerant response, whose symptoms typically include headaches, skin complaints, watery eyes, nasal congestion and irritable bowel syndrome.

Antigens, which provoke the allergic response and the creation of antibodies, are usually proteins or simple substances that combine with or modify the body's own proteins. The antigen may be a product containing proteins, such as some laundry detergents. House dust, pollen and animal hairs are all derived from proteins. More obvious are the proteins in food, like meat, cheese, milk and mushrooms. Wheatgerm oil (a vegetable oil), for instance, is protein based and best avoided by people suffering from allergies.

As they are not protein based, essential oils will not cause an allergic reaction. However, it is possible to be intolerant or hypersensitive to essential oils, especially those that have been adulterated or mixed with a solvent. If you think you are intolerant to a specific oil, check that it is a pure, distilled oil since you may well be reacting to the solvent rather than to the oil itself.

People can be intolerant to almost anything, from coffee to perfumes. This seems to be an increasingly frequent phenomenon. It has been suggested that the growing amount of additives, preservatives and coloring in food products, as well as the increasing number of chemicals used in their cultivation, are making people more intolerant.

For those who are hypersensitive, it is best to first test a drop of the chosen essential oil on the forearm to see if there is any reaction after eight hours. This is known as a *patch test*.

When a person suddenly becomes intolerant to a substance they have used for years, we say they have become *sensitized*. The aldehyde content, for example, in some essential oils makes them *sensitizers*. Once you are sensitized to an oil, you will normally react to any oil containing the component that caused the sensitization in the first place. I have seen this reaction suddenly occur with people using a yarrow oil (*Achillea millefolium*), which contains a large amount of aldehydes.

Some oils with a furocoumarin content are phototoxic. In other words, they make the skin more sensitive to sunlight, so it is best not to sunbathe for an hour after using them. This group of oils is formed mainly from the citrus group, and a few exceptions like angelica (*Angelica archangelica*).

It is always wise to err on the side of caution and follow recommended guidelines when using essential oils for healing at home. But as long as you treat essential oils with the respect they deserve, there is no need to be concerned.

5

CHEMISTRY
AND BOTANY

———

In order to use essential oils safely and effectively it is helpful to have some understanding of what they consist of and the plants from which they originate. A basic knowledge of the chemistry and botany involved, or just an overview of their importance, can help guard against the indiscriminate and random use of essential oils.

You can cook dinner without being a food scientist but a little knowledge about food values and groupings can go a long way toward making the meal a nutritionally balanced one. In the same way, knowing the chemical composition of each essential oil will give you a good indication of both its hazardous and helpful effects. Likewise, to be able to classify the plants from which the oils are derived is useful because a pattern emerges whereby certain therapeutic trends are shown to be characteristic of certain plant families.

I will restrict the scientific information to a minimum, providing just enough data to show you how and why the contents of these tiny glass bottles can have the potential to heal — or to harm if misused.

Chemistry

Carbon, hydrogen and oxygen are the building blocks of life and are contained in all essential oils. They combine to form molecular structures that can be grouped into families of chemicals.

Chemical Families

The main chemical families we will be dealing with are: acids and esters, alcohols, aldehydes, ketones, lactones, oxides, phenols and terpenes. The chemical constituents of each family have a characteristic molecular structure and tend to have similar pharmacological effects, whether they are analgesic, anti-inflammatory, sedative or so on.

We can now skate through the most common chemical families, learn to recognize some examples of their members by their distinctive suffix and note their main effects.

Acids and Esters

Organic acids rarely exist on their own in essential oils and only in small amounts. They combine with an alcohol to form esters, which commonly end in *-ate*, e.g. *linalyl acetate*. They are calming and tonic in their effect, anti-inflammatory, antifungal, encourage the formation of scar tissue and reduce muscle spasm. These qualities make them particularly useful for treating skin complaints. Lavender (*Lavandula angustifolia* and *L. vera*) is the best known example of an essential oil with a high ester content.

Alcohols

These end in *-ol*, e.g. *eucalyptol* and are stimulating and strongly bactericidal in their effect. Essential oils that contain alcohols are good for treating children because they are generally non-toxic and do not irritate the skin. You can safely use German chamomile (*Matricaria chamomilla*) on small children and babies.

ALDEHYDES

They either end in -*al* or have the word *aldehyde* in their name, e.g. *citral* or *cinnamic aldehyde*. Aldehydes are useful hypotensives that calm the nervous system by lowering blood pressure, and are also good anti-inflammatories. In addition, they are cooling because they cause dilation of the veins, and are antiviral. If used carelessly, however, they can sensitize the skin, causing a rash in some people that will reappear every time an oil containing an aldehyde is used. Cinnamon bark (*Cinnamomum zeylanicum*) and lemongrass (*Cymbopogon citratus*) both have a high aldehyde content.

KETONES

They usually end in -*one*, e.g. *menthone*. There are greater variations in the structure of ketones and thus the workings of members of this family. They generally sedate, heal wounds (by encouraging the formation of scar tissue) and break down mucus and fat. Some variations have been found to be expectorant, stimulant, anti-inflammatory, analgesic and anticoagulant in their effects.

Ketones are also considered neurotoxic (toxic to the nervous system), although this seems to depend on the precise form of ketone present. For example, there are differences in the structure and therefore the effect of thujone (present in a species of thyme — e.g. *Thymus vulgaris* ct thujanol-4) and carvone (present in caraway — *Carum carvi*). Until more research is done and unless you are an experienced practitioner, it is safest not to use oils containing high amounts of ketones on pregnant women, babies or epileptics. These include sage (*Salvia officinalis*), hyssop (*Hyssopus officinalis*) and aniseed (*Pimpinella anisum*).

LACTONES

Because the molecules of this chemical grouping are too large to come through distillation, they are present only in expressed oils — the citrus group. Lactones are cooling, and break down and expel mucus. Coumarins, the largest members of this group, are uplifting in their effect, though they can be sedative and are hypotensive. Furocoumarins are known for the photosensitivity they induce. After using oils like bergamot (*Citrus bergamia*) or orange (*Citrus aurantium*), containing large amounts of these, it is best not to sunbathe for a couple of hours.

OXIDES

Opinion is divided about the difference between oxides and phenols, so they should be approached as cautiously as you would a phenol. Although oxides are rare, 1,8 cineole or eucalyptol is commonly used because it is contained in eucalyptus oil (*Eucalyptus globulus*). This oxide efficiently breaks down mucus, relieving coughs, colds and respiratory congestion. However, it is a skin irritant.

PHENOLS

Like alcohols these end in -*ol*. To avoid any confusion with alcohols, their names simply have to be learned. The most common ones are *carvacrol*, *eugenol* and *thymol*. They are very powerful germ-fighting agents, stimulating to both the nervous and the immune systems, but can be irritating to the skin and toxic to the liver. Essential oils containing phenols should not be overused in either frequency or quantity. For example, clove oil (*Syzygium aromaticum*) relieves specific localized conditions such as a toothache, but should not be swallowed.

TERPENES

Terpenes, because of their chemical structure, have hardly any aroma but are present in almost all essential oils. They have the ending *-ene* — e.g. *pinene* and *phellandrene* — and are considered to be antiseptic, bactericidal, antiviral, analgesic and stimulating to the immune system. Perhaps their most important action is as quenchers: their presence is thought to dilute or "quench" the more irritant effects of other chemicals in the oil.

Technological advances have made it possible to identify some of the molecules that make up essential oils. But there are still many undetected components within these complex chemical structures and their effects remain unknown. Nevertheless, the essential oil trade is beginning to list those known and researched constituents present in their oils so that users can place them into their chemical families and have some guidance as to their likely pharmacological effect.

CHEMICAL VARIABILITY

Growers and suppliers find it difficult to provide exact information about the quantity of each of the main components contained in an oil. Changes in the soil, the climate and when the crop is harvested mean that no chemical will be present in the same proportions at each distillation.

Controlling the growing conditions can reduce these variations. However, since the presence of some constituents can vary from 20 to 70 percent, a sample of each distillation should be analyzed to determine its contents. Readings can be taken by a gas-liquid chromatograph. Traders argue that this expensive method is not foolproof, while consumers increasingly want to know what they are buying.

It must be said, however, that there is no direct and simple connection between the individual constituents of an essential oil and its overall effects. The make-up of an oil is intricate; it is more than the sum of its parts. The different chemicals work together to produce a set of effects that often differ from their individual indications.

These complications also explain why a synthetic oil cannot be a substitute for a true essential oil. An aroma can be reconstituted to make a perfume, or a chemical can be isolated to make a drug, but the therapeutic action of an essential oil owes more than we have yet defined to the complex synergy of its chemical components.

Until there has been more research we can only use the knowledge of what has been uncovered about the chemistry of essential oils as a general guide to their possible effects.

BOTANY

All plants are classified into botanical families according to their similarities. There are around twenty families with some two hundred plants that produce essential oils. Not all of these are suitable for aromatherapy; some are used only by the food or fragrance industry.

PLANT FAMILIES

The botanical family names are of Latin derivation and end in *-aceae*, e.g. *Rutaceae* or *Lauraceae*. Botanical families are plant groups and, just as we would expect members of a human family to have similar physical characteristics, so members of the same plant family share the same structural characteristics. For example, all the members of the Umbelliferae family have the same umbrella-shaped flower heads.

In the same way, the essential oil that comes from each botanical family seems to have common physiological effects on people. For example, the Myrtaceae family includes all the eucalypti, such as *Melaleuca alternifolia* (tea tree), *Melaleuca leucadendron* (cajuput) and *Myrtus communis* (myrtle). The essential oils derived from these plants are all known respiratory decongestants and are highly anti-infectious. The digestive properties of the Umbelliferae family—e.g. *Carum carvi* (caraway), *Angelica archangelica* (angelica) and *Coriandrum sativum* (coriander)—are also well documented.

The following is an alphabetical list of the main families with some examples of the plants they contain. The therapeutic trends shown by most of the essential oils in each family are also given. As already stated, it is useful to recognize the botanical family to which a plant belongs because the healing characteristics of a family are carried by its family members.

Just as gardeners have to take care to identify a type of plant by using the generic and specific names if they want to grow a particular color, texture, shape or size, when you choose an essential oil you must clarify the botanical family and the plant from which it comes if you want to be sure of its aroma and likely therapeutic actions.

GENUS

Each plant family may have several members grouped together. The name of the group, or genus, can be considered like a person's surname — Chun, Smith, etc. Hence *Lavandula* is the botanical "surname" for the genus to which the different varieties of lavender belong.

SPECIES

In order to differentiate between plants in the same genus we give them the equivalent of a first name, such as *Lavandula angustifolia* for a particular species of lavender. This identifies the species within the genus.

THE IMPORTANCE OF LATIN NAMES

It is necessary to refer to plants and their oils by their Latin names — to be as specific as possible when identifying a species of oil — in order to be sure of what you are buying. You should be aware that a number of different plants can have the same common name, for example *Anthemis nobilis* and *Matricaria chamomilla* are popularly known as chamomile. On the other hand, a single genus may have more

Family	Essential Oil	Indication
Annonaceae	ylang ylang *(Cananga odorata)*	calming, hypotensive
Burseraceae	frankincense *(Boswellia carteri),* myrrh *(Commiphora myrrha)*	expectorant, wound healing
Compositae	German chamomile *(Matricaria chamomilla),* marigold *(Tagetes minuta)*	anti-inflammatory, soothing to the skin and digestive system
Cupressaceae	cypress *(Cupressus sempervirens),* juniper berry *(Juniperus communis)*	astringent, diuretic
Geraniaceae	geranium *(Pelargonium graveolens)*	antiseptic, calming, soothing to the skin
Labiatae	clary sage *(Salvia sclarea),* European basil *(Ocimum basilicum),* hyssop *(Hyssopus officinalis),* lavender *(Lavandula angustifolia),* peppermint *(Mentha x piperita),* rosemary *(Rosmarinus officinalis),* sage *(Salvia officinalis),* thyme *(Thymus vulgaris)*	anti-inflammatory, decongestant, stimulating (except lavender), tonic
Lauraceae	cinnamon bark *(Cinnamomum zeylanicum),* rosewood *(Aniba rosaeodora)*	antifungal, antiviral, bactericidal, tonic

Family	Essential Oil	Indication
Myrtaceae	clove *(Syzygium aromaticum)*, eucalyptus *(Eucalyptus globulus)*, myrtle *(Myrtus communis)*, niaouli *(Melaleuca viridiflora)*, tea tree *(Melaleuca alternifolia)*	anti-infectious, especially of the respiratory tract, stimulant, tonic
Pinaceae	cedarwood *(Cedrus atlantica)*, pine *(Pinus sylvestris)*	anticatarrhal, antiseptic
Piperaceae	black pepper *(Piper nigrum)*	analgesic, anticatarrhal
Ruataceae	bergamot *(Citrus bergamia)*, lemon *(Citrus limon)*, lime *(Citrus medica var. vulgaris)*, neroli *(Citrus aurantium var. amara)*, orange *(Citrus aurantium)*	reducing muscle spasm
Umbelliferae	aniseed *(Pimpinella anisum)*, caraway *(Carum carvi)*, coriander *(Coriandrum sativum)*, fennel *(Foeniculum vulgare)*	digestive, uterine stimulant
Zingiberaceae	ginger *(Zingiber officinale)*	anticatarrhal, digestive, tonic, warming

than one common name. The *Juniperus* can be everything from a Texan or Virginian cedarwood to a savin or a plain juniper.

This is why it is essential not to be content with a bottle simply labeled "lavender." Only the Latin generic name with its species and any other divisions can prevent the confusion of one plant with another. If we consider that *Lavandula stoechas* contains up to 70 percent ketones (which are neurotoxic and should be used with care), while *Lavandula vera* is relatively gentle, the importance of being precise about the plant from which the oil originates becomes clear. It is not good enough to say you want lavender without stating precisely which one!

Although many of the bottles of oil sold in the stores are still not labeled with this information, many of the mail-order suppliers are now listing the botanical details of the plants from which their oils are distilled.

MORE SUBDIVISIONS

There are further groupings below the level of species such as geographical location or cross-fertilization. These divisions may or may not be reflected by changes in appearance of the plant, but the chemical composition and the therapeutic effects of the essential oil it yields will definitely vary.

The following is a list of these junior divisions and their abbreviations, which you are likely to find on a retail or trade list.

VARIETIES

A *variety* indicates an important subdivision of a species. Species often have several closely related varieties. The name is usually in Latin and written, for example, *Foeniculum vulgare* var. *dulce* (sweet fennel).

CULTIVARS

If the variety has evolved through cultivation rather than in the wild, then it is called a *cultivar*. The name is usually not in Latin and often comes from the person who cultivated the particular type. It is written, for instance, *Pinus strobus* "Nana" (a type of pine).

CHEMOTYPES

These are probably the most relevant to aromatologists. They refer to plants that are visually the same but produce chemically different essential oils. Many plants have several chemotypes that occur naturally. Thyme is a good example, and might be written *Thymus vulgaris* ct linalool. The abbreviation *ct* refers to the chemotype, while the alcohol written at the end (in this case linalool) refers to the main chemical constituent present in the chemotype.

HYBRIDS

These have genetically distinct parents. The parent plants may be different cultivars, varieties, species or genera but are not from different families. The word *hybrida* or an *x* will often appear in the title, e.g. *Mentha x piperita* (peppermint).

WHY DO PLANTS PRODUCE ESSENTIAL OILS?

Essential oils are a product of a plant's secondary metabolism, which also produces the larger molecular structures that form tannins, steroids, alkaloids, glycosides, bitters, gums and so on. None of these are vital to the plant's survival. *Essential oil* is in fact a misnomer; it is not *essential* to the plant's life like the products of primary metabolism. This process is known as photosynthesis. Here the minerals and water a plant takes from the soil, the carbon dioxide it absorbs from the air and the energy it draws from the sun are turned into glucose, vital for the plant's nourishment and growth.

The exact purpose and function in the plant of the secondary metabolites are not known. They give the plant its flavor and its aroma but there are likely to be several more reasons for their existence. In the case of essential oils some of these may be:

- to ward off bacteria and fungi (they are nature's antiseptics for plants as well as for people)

- to repel insects or other herbivores

- to attract those insects that pollinate plants

- to heal wounds to the plant (as with animals, a plant forms scars)

- to prevent other plants from rooting too close and threatening survival in poor conditions. (A plant can exude camphor and 1,8 cineole that reach the soil and make the conditions too unfriendly for other plants to root.)

- to limit dehydration by forming a vaporous mist of volatile oil around the plant to lessen the water lost from the leaves when conditions are dry. This is most commonly experienced in pine and eucalyptus forests where the air is heavy with the aroma from the essential oils. The Blue Mountains outside Sydney, Australia, have earned their name because of this blue haze that hangs in the air above the thousands of eucalyptuses.

It is worth observing that, although conjectural, many of the justifications for the presence of essential oils in plants are mirrored in the wound-healing, protective, bactericidal and antiseptic uses we are finding for them to safeguard our own health.

However technical, an understanding of the structure and function of plants and the essential oils they contain will illuminate your practice of healing with essential oils.

6

HEALING AT HOME

In this chapter I shall concentrate on ten versatile essential oils and their indications in helping a wide range of simple and common health complaints. These are the oils I use most frequently in treatments and the ones I most recommend for any first-aid kit or bathroom medicine cabinet. If you want to extend your collection, consult the table of essential oils (listed by botanical family) and their therapeutic indications in the previous chapter. Please note, however, that a persistent, inexplicable or complicated problem should not be treated at home without first seeking professional advice.

For safety precautions concerning the mixing, correct quantities, carrier oils, storage and supply, and methods of application please refer to Chapters Four, Eight and Nine.

In the book I specify each of the ten oils by its Latin name. The common name will appear in brackets but should not be relied upon because only the Latin name will direct you to the exact species I am referring to. It is also good to pay special attention to the different species of rosemary, thyme, eucalyptus, juniper berry, cedarwood and chamomile. In the case of lavender, where several (but not all) species are very similar, I have listed together those which can be considered as a group.

Finally, when an oil is denoted *bactericidal*, this is a general guide to its potential. It does not necessarily mean that it has a broad-spectrum antibacterial action as some antibiotics do. On the contrary, certain essential oils have a specific action on named bacteria.

TEN BASIC ESSENTIAL OILS

CARUM CARVI (CARAWAY)

Plant family	Compositae
Parts used	seeds
Main constituents	carvacrol, carvene, carvone, limonene
Properties	anticatarrhal, anti-infectious, digestive and stomachic stimulant
Main country of origin	Holland
Cautions	This oil contains only a trace of the phenolic ether anethole, but there is up to 50 percent carvone, a ketone, present; children and pregnant women would be best advised not to take it.

Indications for Use

This is a good oil for fighting infections of the respiratory and digestive systems. It has also been recommended for treating vertigo.

CITRUS LIMON (LEMON)

Plant family	Rutaceae
Parts used	peel

Main constituents	caprylic acid, citral, geraniol, linalool, limonene, pinene
Properties	bactericidal, calming, cooling
Main country of origin	southern Europe
Cautions	The high terpene content counteracts the effect of citral, an aldehyde, which could otherwise be a skin irritant or sensitizer; be careful not to buy a de-terpented oil.

Indications for Use

Its antiseptic and cleansing properties make this oil good for soothing insect bites, minor skin conditions, boils, verrucas and warts. Because it has a cooling effect, it can help reduce fever. It is also indicated for use as a liver tonic.

EUCALYPTUS GLOBULUS (EUCALYPTUS OR BLUE GUM)

Plant family	Myrtaceae
Parts used	leaves
Main constituents	cineol, eucalyptol, isoborneol, pinene, terpineol
Properties	antifungal, antiviral, bactericidal, breaks down mucus, cooling, expectorant, lowers blood sugar, parasiticidal, pulmonary/urinary antiseptic
Main country of origin	Australia, China, Spain
Cautions	Because of the strong aroma and the oxide 1,8 cineole (eucalyptol) present, it should be used with moderation on small children or people with weak chests; it can also be a skin irritant.

Indications for Use

This oil is renowned for its effectiveness against coughs and colds as a decongestant. It is also a bactericidal. Used as a spray with a 2 percent eucalyptus oil content, it kills 70 percent of ambient staphylococci (according to Jean Valnet, a respected authority in the field). It has been indicated for use in controlling cystitis, intestinal parasites, diabetes, chronic bronchitis, asthma, pneumonia and tuberculosis. In India I found it was prescribed to reduce fever in cases of typhoid, malaria, scarlet fever and measles.

JUNIPERUS COMMUNIS (JUNIPER BERRY)

Plant family	Cupressaceae
Parts used	berries
Main constituents	camphene, campholenic acid, terpineol-4
Properties	antirheumatic, astringent, diuretic, soothing and sedative
Main country of origin	Canada, central and southern Europe, Sweden
Cautions	Because of the diuretic effect, it has been suggested that this oil should not be used in the first few months of pregnancy; however, I have never heard of a miscarriage caused by the controlled use of this oil.

Indications for Use

Its astringency makes this oil good to use on oily skin conditions such as acne. Ulcers—stomach, skin and mouth—and weeping eczema may also respond well. Because it encourages the secretion of uric acids and toxins, it is effective when applied to muscles after sports activities, or in cases of gout, arthritis and rheumatism. It stimulates digestive juices and other secretions of enzymes, making it known as a tonic for digestion. It helps in cases of depletion or debilitation.

LAVANDULA ANGUSTIFOLIA, L. OFFICINALIS, L. VERA (LAVENDER)

Plant family	Labiatae
Parts used	flowering tops, leaves
Main constituents	linalool, linalyl acetate

Properties	antifungal, anti-flammatory, antiseptic, bactericidal, both calming and tonic to the nervous system, reduces scarring
Main country of origin	France, Italy (grown best at high altitude)

Indications for Use

This must be the most frequently used essential oil. A bottle should be kept in every household if only to apply to burns and scalds. Its gentle action makes it safe to use on people of all ages and in all states of health. Because it is calming and sedative, it is frequently suggested for relieving stress, headaches and insomnia. It promotes the healing and prevents the scarring of wounds. It can soothe and cleanse inflamed and dry skin conditions. It assists in the treatment of leg ulcers. As an antiseptic, it is useful in infectious conditions particularly of the chest or upper respiratory tract.

MATRICARIA CHAMOMILLA (GERMAN CHAMOMILE)

Plant family	Compositae
Parts used	flowers
Main constituents	caprylic acid and monylic acid, chamazulene, lamesene
Properties	analgesic, anti-inflammatory, lowers fever through bactericidal action, reduces muscle spasm and relieves nervous irritability, especially in children
Main country of origin	France

Indications for Use

German chamomile essential oil contains a high amount of azulene which is not present in the flowers; it decomposes from a colorless compound during distillation and turns the oil deep blue. This azulene constricts veins and makes a good anti-inflammatory. It can be used to treat both internal and external inflammatory conditions such as gastritis, colitis, cystitis, eczema, leg ulcers and urticaria (nettle rash). I have used it successfully in a case of vulvar pruritus and also find that it relieves the vomiting that often accompanies gastritis, or the biliousness and regurgitation of acid associated with other digestive disorders. Its analgesic effect eases muscular aches and pains, while its ability to reduce muscle spasm is excellent for soothing menstrual and stomach cramps. Hayfever, asthma and many allergic reactions are calmed by its influence.

MELALEUCA ALTERNIFOLIA (TEA TREE)

Plant family	Myrtaceae
Parts used	leaves
Main constituents	1,8 cineole, pinene, terpinen-4-ol
Properties	antifungal, anti-inflammatory, antiviral, bactericidal, stimulating to the immune system
Main country of origin	Australia

Indications for Use

This oil is becoming increasingly popular because of its antiseptic power. It can be applied directly to the skin and is useful in a range of fungal and viral infections, from herpes sores, athlete's foot, ringworm to thrush. Its antiviral properties make it worth trying on all conditions suspected to be of a viral nature such as post-viral syndrome (or ME).

MENTHA X PIPERITA (PEPPERMINT)

Plant family	Labiatae
Parts used	leaves
Main constituents	menthol, menthone
Properties	anti-inflammatory, antiseptic, expectorant, reduces flatulence, nerve stimulant, tonic
Main country of origin	England, France
Cautions	Because of its reputedly high levels of ketones, this oil has been contra-indicated in pregnancy; in fact the ketone pulegone, thought to be abortive, is only

ever present in a small amount or not at all in this oil. It would be prudent to check the ketone content of the oil before buying it, however; many rectified oils are on the market which have a menthone content in excess of 15-30 percent. These should be avoided.

Indications for Use

Peppermint's affinity with the digestive system is becoming well known. The oil can be obtained in tablet form for the relief of irritable bowel syndrome. Indigestion, bad breath — and flatulence can be reduced. Its expectorant quality may aid those suffering from asthma and bronchitis. It can relieve migraines, vertigo, sinusitis and headaches, and I have found that it soothes insect bites and sunburn. As a stimulant it comes into its own for combating general fatigue but if overused can cause insomnia. Jean Valnet suggests its use in cases of scanty or painful menstrual periods.

ROSMARINUS OFFICINALIS (ROSEMARY)→

Plant family	Labiatae
Parts used	flowers, leaves
Main constituents	borneol, camphor, 1,8 cineole, pinene
Properties	antineuralgic, cerebral as well as general stimulant, hypertensive, intestinal and pulmonary antiseptic
Main country of origin	France, Italy, Spain
Cautions	Many chemotypes of this oil are now available; children and pregnant women should not use the verbenone type as this ketone is neurotoxic.

Indications for Use

Being an antiseptic oil, and both a physical and mental stimulant, it can treat fatigue, memory loss, coughs and colds as well as stiff and tired muscles. Debilitating conditions involving pain and weakness benefit the most, whether it be painful periods or fainting and vertigo.

ZINGIBER OFFICINALE (GINGER)

Plant family	Zingiberaceae
Parts used	rhizome
Main constituents	cineol, citral, d-phellandrene, gingerol, isoborneol, zingiberene
Properties	antiseptic, digestive aid, expels mucus and relieves flatulence
Main country of origin	China, Phillipines, Sri Lanka
Cautions	Many chemotypes of this oil are now available; children and pregnant women should not use the verbenone type as this ketone is neurotoxic.

Indications for Use

Ginger is useful in cases where there is a loss of appetite and digestive difficulty, such as nausea, flatulence or constipation. It is antiseptic and warming and helps to remove mucus, which makes it a good choice for bronchial complaints. Rheumatic and muscular conditions, where stiffness and cold are a problem, respond well to ginger oil massage.

CASE AILMENTS FOR HEALING AT HOME WITH THE TEN BASIC ESSENTIAL OILS

A table follows showing the most common problems and my suggestions for helpful oils to use. For quantities and full details on applications, see Chapter Seven. Since I am restricting my recommendations to the ten basic oils as described in this chapter, I will use their common names but please refer back to their correct Latin title before trying any of these examples.

On the whole, applying little and often is the best way to achieve results. For example, taking an inhalation of moderate strength three times a day is better than one super-strong one once a day.

It is best to use a combination of all the oils listed for a complaint rather than one individual oil, except when there is only one oil mentioned.

Complaints	Oil to Use	How to Apply Oils
abscesses	eucalyptus, lavender, tea tree	massage oil, warm compress
athlete's foot	lavender, tea tree	apply directly, drops in a bath
bleeding gums	eucalyptus, lavender, lemon	mouth wash
boils	lavender, tea tree	hot compress
bruises	lavender, rosemary	alternate hot and cold compresses
burns	lavender	apply directly to the affected area. *Note:* first hold the burned area under a cold tap for 15 minutes or until all the stinging is gone
catarrh	caraway, peppermint, rosemary	diffuser, steam inhalation
cellulite	juniper berry, lavender, rosemary	clay application or oil massage
chilblains	ginger, juniper berry, rosemary	massage oil
cold sores	lavender, lemon, tea tree	apply directly, drops in a bath
colds	caraway, eucalyptus, tea tree	diffuser, drops on a tissue, steam inhalation; massage oil applied to sinus area, chest and upper back
constipation	ginger, juniper berry, lemon, rosemary	oil massage in a clockwise direction of skin above the colon

Complaints	Oil to Use	How to Apply Oils
coughs	caraway, eucalyptus, tea tree	massage oil, steam inhalation
cramp	German chamomile, juniper berry, rosemary	massage oil
cuts and abrasions	lavender, tea tree	bathe affected area and apply oils directly on a gauze dressing
cystitis	juniper berry, lavender, tea tree	drops in a bath or a sitz bath
dandruff	rosemary, tea tree	add to shampoo or rinsing water
dermatitis	German chamomile, lavender, tea tree	massage oil, cream or lotion
diaper rash	German chamomile, lavender, tea tree	massage oil, cream or lotion
eczema	German chamomile, lavender, peppermint (weak dilution)	massage oil, cream or lotion
fatigue	ginger, peppermint, rosemary	drops in a bath or inhaled from a tissue
fleas	lemon, tea tree	apply directly, drops in a bath
fluid retention	juniper berry, rosemary	drops in a bath, massage oil
German measles	German chamomile, lavender, tea tree	drops in a bath
gingivitis	German chamomile, eucalyptus, peppermint	mouth wash
hangover	juniper berry, rosemary	drops in a bath, massage oil
hay fever	German chamomile, lemon, peppermint	drops in a bath or inhaled from a tissue

Complaints	Oil to Use	How to Apply Oils
headaches	lavender, peppermint, rosemary	drops in a bath, massage oil applied to neck and shoulders
head lice	tea tree	apply directly in shampoo or rinsing water
heartburn	caraway, eucalyptus, peppermint	massage oil applied to abdominal area
heat rash/ bumps	lavender, peppermint	drops in a bath, massage oil, cream or lotion
hemorrhoids	lemon, tea tree	drops in a sitz bath
hiccups	lavender, lemon	inhale drops from a tissue
indigestion	German chamomile, ginger, peppermint	massage oil applied to abdominal area
influenza	caraway, eucalyptus, peppermint	drops in a bath, massage oil, steam inhaltion
insect bites	German chamomile, lavender, peppermint	apply lavender directly; mix other two oils into a cream or gel
insomnia	lavender	drops in a bath; put several drops on your pillow or add to a room diffuser
laryngitis	lavender, tea tree	gargle
mouth ulcers	lemon, peppermint, tea tree	mouth wash
muscular aches and pains	ginger, lavender, rosemary	massage oil
nausea	lavender, peppermint	inhale drops from a tissue

Complaints	Oil to Use	How to Apply Oils
neuralgia	lavender, peppermint	massage oil
ringworm	lemon, tea tree	apply drops mixed in lotion, cream or gel
scalds (see burns)		
shingles	lavender, tea tree	drops in a bath, massage lotion
shock	lavender, lemon	inhale drops from a tissue
sinusitis	eucalyptus, peppermint, rosemary	massage oil applied to sinus area of the face, steam inhalation
sore throat (see laryngitis)		
sprains	German chamomile, lavender, rosemary	apply in alternate hot and cold compresses
stiffness	ginger, lavender, rosemary	massage oil or gel
sunburn	lavender, peppermint	lotion or cream
thrush	lavender, tea tree	drops in a sitz bath
urticaria	German chamomile, lavender	drops in a bath, massage oil, lotion or cream, warm compress
varicose veins	lavender, rosemary	massage oil or lotion. *Note:* to avoid pushing blood into the vein, never massage the skin on or below the vein; always between the heart and the vein
warts	tea tree	apply directly to the wart

7

HEALING METHODS

There are many ways to use essential oils at home. As well as using the oils individually, you can mix them together or combine them with carrier oils to create treatments suitable for a wide range of conditions, whether the cause is physiological or psychological.

Essential oils enter the body by the following routes:

- absorption through the skin in combination with a carrier oil, lotion, cream, gel, clay mix or water

- inhalation through the nose and mouth with air and steam

The basic essential oils listed in chapters Five and Six are suitable for use according to the methods and in the quantities suggested here. Please see these chapters for the botanical terms and note that *Lavandula angustifolia* is intended wherever "lavender" is specified in a recipe.

CARRIERS

Apart from *Melaleuca alternifolia* (tea tree) and *Lavandula officinalis* (lavender), which can be applied directly to the skin, all essential oils should first be mixed with or carried by another medium. They are too strong and too concentrated to be used directly.

Air, water, steam, alcohol, oil, lotion or cream are used to dilute, disperse and then carry the essential oil into the body. Essential oils can penetrate the skin or enter through any orifice, i.e., nose, mouth, anus or vagina.

SKIN ABSORPTION

We tend to think of our skin as a waterproof, protective coating that keeps things out. Many of my clients believe that essential oils can go no farther than skin deep until I explain the penetrative ability of the oils. The aromatic molecules making up essential oils are far smaller and more soluble in fatty tissue than those found in most other substances — including vegetable oils, which tend to stay on the surface of the skin because their molecules are too large to pass through the dermal cells.

Help in clearing up this misconception about skin penetration has actually come from innovations in traditional medical treatments: the use of hormone replacement therapy, for instance, as well as nicotine patches and the introduction of painkilling gels such as Ibuprofen. These have all helped to spread the acceptance that certain substances can be absorbed through the skin.

Because the skin is the largest organ of the body, one advantage of a full body massage with essential oils is that a large surface area is covered, allowing a large amount of oil to penetrate. The tiny molecules of an essential oil enter through the hair follicles and sweat glands; being fat soluble, the oil can also seep through the fatty area between skin cells. The small blood capillaries lying below the top layers of the skin then take the oil to circulate in the bloodstream around the body. Through the testing of exhaled air and urine it has been shown that essential oils enter the body very quickly after being rubbed into the skin.

INHALATION

The inhalation of essential oils can influence our mood and stimulate our memory. It can also evoke a physical response in the same way that the smell of a favorite food can make you salivate. When they are inhaled, the molecules of an essential oil are detected by cells in the nose that are designed to react to a specific aroma. Since not everyone has all of these receptor cells, there are certain odors that some of us cannot smell. However, a message is sent directly to the brain in response to a smell, whether you are aware of it or not. The part of the brain which analyzes the smell is also the part that is responsible for our emotional and memory responses — hence the emotional or physical response to an evocative smell.

After breathing in the oils through the nose or the mouth, a certain amount will permeate the mucus membrane and enter the lungs. This is why oils such as eucalyptus, rosemary and lavender play a valuable role in treating conditions of the upper respiratory tract and chest, such as colds, sinusitis, headaches and some forms of asthma.

The safest methods for healing with essential oils at home are those that involve entry through the skin or nose. Internal ingestion, whether orally or by using suppositories or pessaries, is more hazardous and should only be carried out under supervision.

Methods of Application

Baths

Soaking for ten minutes or so in a bath containing an essential oil offers dual benefits: it will be inhaled through your nose and absorbed through your skin.

Run a warm bath and when it is full add 8 drops in total of up to 4 essential oils of your choice. Halve this number for children and the elderly, halve it again for toddlers, and halve it again for babies. Add the oils once the bath is full and swish the water around to encourage them to disperse. A single droplet could sting you if you sat on it!

Essential oils are not fully soluble in water, so you may want to mix them with a substance containing fat, such as oil or milk. Milk is often the preferred option for a baby's bath. The disadvantage of mixing them with a vegetable oil is that it can leave a greasy ring around your tub; your skin, however, benefits from the softening and moisturizing effect of the vegetable oil.

It is now possible to buy bath dispersants for essential oils from some mail-order companies. These are vegetable-derived, natural emulsifiers that, when mixed with essential oils, allow them to disperse fully in water.

Recipe for Relaxation

geranium	2 drops
lavender	4 drops
orange	2 drops

Recipe for Revitalization

lemon	4 drops
peppermint	2 drops
rosemary	2 drops

Recipe for Soothing Aches and Pains

black pepper	2 drops
juniper berry	2 drops
lavender	2 drops
rosemary	2 drops

CLAY

The minerals and trace elements found in clay are beneficial in their own right. Clay's astringent and detoxifying properties make it useful for drawing impurities from the skin. In turn the drawing action can stimulate local blood supply and increase the effect of the essential oils mixed with it.

Mix essential oils with clay in the same proportions as for vegetable oils (see under *Massage*). Add them to dry powder and mix with enough floral or spring water to make a paste. Once you obtain the desired consistency, you can apply the paste to the area to be treated and leave it on for 10 to 15 minutes.

Clay packs are commonly used in hair treatments and as face packs for oily skin.

Recipe for Treating Acne

clay	10 mg
bergamot	1 drop
tea tree	1 drop

Recipe for Treating Dry Skin

clay	10 mg
German chamomile	2 drops

Recipe for Treating Oily Skin

clay	10 mg
lavender	1 drop
tea tree	1 drop

COMPRESSES

Compresses can be applied either hot or cold. To prepare a compress, soak a piece of absorbent, cotton cloth in a bowl of boiled and then cooled water. To every half-pint of water add 8 drops of the selected oil or combination of oils (see recipes below). Squeeze the cloth and put it on the area of the body to be treated. For hot compresses you can place a hot water bottle on top; for cold compresses you can place a bag of frozen peas or a medical freezer bag on top. Each compress should be left on for 10 minutes. The treatment can be repeated 3 to 4 times a day, if necessary.

A hot compress is best for treating dull pain or stiffness, while a cold one is good for inflammation. For sprains and bruises, alternate hot and cold compresses using hyssop, lavender and rosemary oils to help reduce the swelling. A compress using German chamomile and lavender oils is useful for treating stomach and head pain. For boils and insect bites, use peppermint and German chamomile. Some arthritic pain, accompanied by inflammation, responds well to a mixture of juniper berry, lavender and German chamomile.

Recipe for Clearing Head Colds

German chamomile	4 drops
lavender	4 drops

Recipe for Easing Stiff Joints

black pepper	4 drops
German chamomile	4 drops

Recipe for Reducing Inflammation

German chamomile	4 drops
juniper berry	4 drops

Recipe for Treating Boils, Insect Bites

lavender	4 drops
tea tree	4 drops

Recipe for Treating Headaches

eucalyptus	6 drops
peppermint	2 drops

DIFFUSERS AND VAPORIZERS

Many of these are now available for use with essential oils. They range from the simple pottery burner used with a night light to an electrically powered unit. The vapors released after heating contain the chosen essential oil and are diffused into the atmosphere.

Diffusers with pine or lemon oil are a good way to deodorize the atmosphere. Some people with allergies to house dust, mites or pollen find the effect of these antiseptic or calming oils released into the atmosphere very helpful. In a sickroom they can have an anti-infectious or bactericidal effect, depending on the oil you choose. In the case of head colds, a decongestant or expectorant oil such as eucalyptus or rosemary discharged into the room throughout the night can offer relief. A sedative oil such as lavender may aid sleep.

Essential oils should be used undiluted or added to water, depending on the variety of diffuser you are using. They should never be mixed with a vegetable oil in this situation. The number of drops you use depends on how long you want the oil to burn and how large an area you want to cover. Manufacturers of some electric diffusers recommend that you run them for 15 minutes every two hours.

Because essential oils are highly flammable, I prefer electric diffusers. Anything that uses a bare flame like a candle or night light introduces the risk of the oil coming into contact with a direct heat source. For this reason I am also cautious about the use of light-bulb rings that fit around the top of a light bulb. If you do use these, the essential oil should only be put in the ring when the bulb is cold and the light is switched off.

A less expensive method of creating a room vaporizer is to put a small towel soaked in warm water mixed with some drops of essential oil over a hot radiator. This works beautifully during the winter.

DIRECT INHALATION

One or 2 drops of essential oil on a handkerchief, tissue or pillow, which can be sniffed whenever needed, has a stimulating or calming effect depending on the oil chosen. Whether you are studying for exams, driving long distances or simply feeling weary, inhalation of an oil such as rosemary is a convenient way to perk yourself up. Equally, using vetiver can be calming in a tense situation, such as before an interview; lavender can relax you to sleep.

HAND AND FOOT BATHS

Fill a bowl with hot water, adding one of the recipes listed below and soaking the hand or foot for 10 minutes 3 to 4 times a day, depending on the condition being treated. For children, start with only 1 drop of the recipe you are using.

Recipe for Easing Sprains

lavender	3 drops
rosemary	3 drops

Recipe for Reducing Bruising

hyssop	2 drops
lavender	4 drops

Recipe for Soothing Eczema

German chamomile	3 drops
lavender	3 drops

GARGLES

For sore throats, 2 to 3 drops of a soothing and anti-infectious oil, such as tea tree or lavender, mixed into a glass of water can offer relief and fight infection before it reaches the chest. Before each gargle, stir the water since essential oils are not soluble in water. Repeat twice a day and do not swallow.

JACUZZIS

These offer the best way of using essential oils in a bath. The movement of the water disperses the oils very effectively, which reduces the problem of the oils sitting on the surface of the water and not penetrating the skin.

It is advisable not to use essential oils mixed with a vegetable oil in a jacuzzi because the vegetable oil may clog and damage the pump. (See "Baths" above for recipes.)

MASSAGE

VEGETABLE OILS   These are the most commonly used carriers for applying essential oils to the skin. Mineral oil, which is often used for babies, is not suitable because it does not easily absorb the essential oils and tends to sit on the skin. There are a variety of vegetable oils, all with their own therapeutic properties (for more details see the next chapter). Always buy cold-pressed vegetable oils because this is the only production method that avoids contamination from any chemical processing.

Vegetable oils are fatty, and because essential oils are fat soluble, they blend well together. Vegetable oils fix or hold the volatile essential oils so that they can soak into the skin. Once mixed, the oils can be self-applied to a specific area of the body or given in a full or partial body massage. Vegetable oils are excellent for massage because they allow the therapist's hands to glide across the skin.

The proportion of essential oil to vegetable oil is usually 2 to 3 percent for adults (halve this quantity for children, and halve it again for babies). Twenty drops of essential oil make roughly 5 ml. The ratio works out to:

- 1 drop of essential oil to every 2 ml of carrier oil
- 5 drops of essential oil to every 10 ml of carrier oil

Try not to blend more than you need for one application since the mixture will oxidize and lose its therapeutic value. (See the section at the end of this chapter on blending and storing larger amounts.)

The total quantity depends on the area you are going to cover. A full body massage normally takes between 10 and 15 ml of oil, depending on the size and the weight of the person, the dryness of the skin and the amount of body hair.

Recipe for Reducing Stretch Marks

peach kernel oil	8 ml
rose hip oil	2 ml
neroli	5 drops

Recipe for Treating Varicose Veins

sunflower oil	8 ml
St. John's wort oil	2 drops
lavender	2 drops
lemon	3 drops

Note: Do not massage directly over a varicose vein.

Massage can be an excellent way of relieving conditions that have an emotional and psychological aspect:

Recipe for Dispelling Lethargy

sunflower oil	10 ml
juniper berry	2 drops
rosemary	2 drops

Recipe for Relieving Premenstrual Syndrome (PMS)

almond oil	10 ml
clary sage	1 drop
fennel	2 drops
geranium	1 drop

Recipe for Relieving Stress/Tension

apricot oil	10 ml
lavender	2 drops
ylang ylang	3 drops

Recipe for Treating Depression

almond oil	8 ml
geranium	2 drops
bergamot	3 drops

Recipe for Treating Insomnia

almond oil	8 ml
lime blossom oil	2 drops
bergamot	2 drops
lavender	3 drops

LOTIONS AND CREAMS   Lotions and creams have the advantage of being less greasy than vegetable oils and often soak more quickly into the skin. Add essential oils in the same proportion as you would for mixing with a vegetable oil (see above).

Natural, non-fragrant lotions and creams suitable for carrying essential oils are available from many mail-order suppliers (see "Helpful Addresses" in the back of this book). Some of these can be supplemented by mixing in vegetable oils or floral waters. The most convenient types are manufactured in such a way that you can add essential oils without using heat for blending.

For self-application, lotions and creams are convenient as they rub in easily and do not stain or discolor clothing, unlike oil blends. Creams are usually best suited to hand or face treatments.

Recipe for Moisturizing Dry Skin

lotion	7 ml
evening primrose oil	3 ml
geranium	5 drops

Recipe for Treating Bruises

lotion	7 ml
arnica oil	3 ml
lavender	3 drops
rosemary	2 drops

Recipe for Treating Cuts and Abrasions

lotion	7 ml
mullein oil	3 ml
lavender	3 drops

GELS   Gel-based materials derived from natural polysaccharides (do not use petroleum-based gels as these are composed of mineral rather than organic compounds) are less oily than vegetable oils, creams and lotions. This means that they are less slippery and easier to apply where using a cream or oil could be awkward, such as someone with arthritic hands. As with lotions and creams, gels leave no oil stains on clothing. (Like lotions and creams, these are available from mail-order suppliers.)

Recipe for Easing Stiff Joints

gel	10 ml
caraway	3 drops
lavender	3 drops

Recipe for Treating Sinusitis

gel	10 ml
black pepper	1 drop
eucalyptus	1 drop

MOUTH WASHES

Prepare the oils in the same way as for a gargle (see above). Swish the water around in the mouth and do not swallow. Mouth washes can be useful for treating bleeding gums, tooth decay and mouth ulcers, and after dental surgery. For these cases 2 to 3 drops of either lemon, lavender, eucalyptus or tea tree oil, or a combination of these, can help. This treatment is best carried out after every meal when the teeth have been cleaned.

Recipe for Soothing Toothache

water	150 ml
clove	1 drop

Recipe for Treating Mouth Ulcers

water	150 ml
tea tree	2 drops

SAUNAS

Sitting in dry or wet steam rooms is a wonderful way to clear the head. Decongestion can be aided by adding 2 to 3 drops of pine or thyme oil to the water that is ladled over the coals in a sauna.

SHAMPOOS

Essential oils can be added to shampoos to enhance treatments for dandruff and dry or oily hair. Use the same proportions as for vegetable oils (see under "Massage").

SITZ BATHS

Sitz baths can be used to treat thrush, stitches after childbirth, vaginal itching and hemorrhoids. Only 3 to 4 drops of tea tree, lavender or lemon (or a combination of these, totalling 4 drops) are necessary in each bath taken 3 to 4 times a day to alleviate the discomfort, itching or inflammation associated with the above complaints. Tea tree oil will also fight the yeast-like fungus that causes thrush.

Recipe for Aiding Vaginal Healing after Childbirth

lavender	6 drops

Recipe for Controlling Thrush

lavender	3 drops
tea tree	3 drops

Recipe for Soothing Hemorrhoids

lavender	3 drops
lemon	3 drops

STEAM INHALATION

To a bowl containing half a pint of almost boiling water add 3 drops of essential oils. Put a towel over your head and breathe deeply, keeping your eyes shut to avoid any stinging. Continue for 3 to 5 minutes. Little and often is a good rule to observe when you are using inhalations. It is better to repeat the treatment up to 4 times a day rather than increase the number of drops at each sitting.

Recipe for Relieving Colds

caraway	1 drop
eucalyptus	1 drop
lavender	1 drop

When treating children for colds, make up the mixture in a small bottle and start with only 1 drop for each treatment since the aroma may be too overpowering.

Recipe for Treating Asthmatics

lavender	1 drop
pine	1 drop

All of the oils in both of these recipes, plus peppermint, are excellent for treating colds, catarrh, sinusitis, coughs and chest infections. In addition to relieving congestion, they fight infection and break down mucus.

TREATING DANDRUFF AND HEAD LICE

A blend of any vegetable oil with rosemary or tea tree essential oils can be applied to the scalp for the treatment of such conditions as dandruff or head lice. Warm 20 ml of vegetable oil, then add 10 drops of rosemary or tea tree oil, or 5 of each. Massage the mixture in for 10 minutes and then leave it on for an hour. During this time a hot towel should be wrapped around the head because the increase in temperature will help the absorption of the oil. Finally, rub shampoo into the hair and scalp before washing off with warm water and rubbing dry. Repeat every other night for a week, if necessary.

PREPARING AND KEEPING LARGER AMOUNTS OF OIL BLENDS

If you know that you want to repeat a treatment several times, it is easier to mix a larger amount of the oil, lotion or cream. To do this you need to take measures to preserve the blend.

For mixing oils you need a bottle made of dark-brown glass. Such bottles are available from any health food store and come in varying sizes. I will give a recipe for making up a 100 ml bottle of blended oil. This measure can be adjusted as long as the ratios of the ingredients remain the same.

Count in 40 to 50 drops of your chosen essential oil or oils into the glass bottle. Then add 5 to 10 percent (5 to 10 ml) wheatgerm oil — this acts as a natural preservative, prolonging the lifetime of the mix. Finally, fill the bottle with your chosen vegetable oil. If you are using a heavy oil or a specialist oil such as avocado or rose hip, it is better to add only 20 ml and fill the rest of the bottle with a lighter vegetable oil such as sunflower oil. Remember to shake the oil mix well before using.

Label the bottle clearly, indicating its contents, its purpose and the date it was mixed. Do not keep it longer than necessary and certainly for no longer than six months.

The same method applies to mixing larger amounts of a lotion or cream. Here it is important to add the vegetable and essential oils gradually, shaking or stirring all the time.

PREPARING AND KEEPING LARGER AMOUNTS OF PURE ESSENTIAL OILS

If you find that a certain mixture of pure essential oils is suited for the condition you wish to treat, and you plan to repeat the treatment several times, you can fill a 10 ml dark-brown bottle with your chosen oils.

For example, if you are using 3 drops of lavender to 3 drops of eucalyptus to 4 drops of lemon to treat a head cold, put 3 ml each of lavender and eucalyptus, together with 4 ml of lemon, into one 10 ml bottle. (Use the rough guide of 20 drops to 1 ml.) The mix is now ready to use each time you need it.

A mixture of true essential oils may be kept in a dark-brown bottle with a screw top in a cool place for up to two years.

DOSAGE

In describing the above methods of use, I have recommended a dosage in terms of a number of drops of essential oils. Since these are not standardized, the size of the drops can vary. Only in France, where drops are normally measured with a calibrated pipette, can quantities be exact. It is therefore advisable to choose the lowest dosage suggested in this and other books on the subject.

It must be said, however, that given the small amounts of oil, and the gentle methods of application described above, a variation between a drop or two should not cause too much concern.

8

USING VEGETABLE AND MACERATED OILS

There is a whole range of vegetable and infused or macerated herbal oils that you can use in conjunction with essential oils. Previously a vegetable oil was used simply to carry the essential oil into the body. Now aromatologists are recognizing that some of these carrier oils have a therapeutic value in their own right. They can also complement the healing effect of essential oils: they are not just carriers.

VEGETABLE OILS

WHAT ARE VEGETABLE OILS?

Vegetable oils are extracted from nuts, seeds or kernels. They are known as *fixed* oils because they are not volatile like essential oils. In other words, they do not evaporate; they are greasy and leave an oily mark on blotting paper.

Because essential oils are fat soluble, vegetable oils are the ideal medium for mixing with them.

They can then penetrate the skin during massage or after any other direct application. A vegetable oil is generally preferred if it is light, not too pungent and cold pressed.

THE COMPONENTS OF VEGETABLE OILS

The precise composition of a vegetable oil varies according to the exact plant and species from which it comes. The extraction process itself will alter the make-up of the oil. Generally vegetable oils consist of fatty acids, lecithin, esters of glycerol, vitamins and minerals. As with essential oils, the therapeutic application of each oil depends on its contents.

HOW VEGETABLE OILS ARE PROCESSED

Cold-pressed extraction from organically grown material produces the finest quality oil for both internal and external use. This process is time consuming and costly, however, and there is only a small specialist market for cold-pressed oils, which further inflates prices.

The food industry usually settles for hot extraction, which can change the nature of an oil. Although this process is more complicated, the yield is greater than that achieved by cold pressing. This kind of processing often includes refining the oil still further to increase its stability, thereby prolonging its shelf life. For example, the fatty acids that are prone to oxidation are removed to prevent rancidity. But vital nutrients such as vitamins are destroyed, making these oils unsuitable for therapeutic treatment.

Despite its name, a low level of heat is used in cold pressing — just enough to help release the oil from the nuts, seeds or kernels. The first oil to be expressed is known as the *virgin* oil. Even if heat is generated naturally from the force involved in squeezing out the oil, it is carefully monitored in order not to exceed a stipulated level.

PURCHASING AND QUALITY CONTROL

Vegetable oils are perishable products and should be bought in small quantities. The problems inherent in storage and instability in virgin, cold-pressed oils mean that some oils like grapeseed are not easily available in this unrefined form. Since the market for high-grade vegetable oils for use in therapy is growing, there are increasing numbers of mail-order companies who can give advice and sell you oils of a quality to use in health care (see "Helpful Addresses").

Risks to be aware of when you choose a vegetable oil are the vast quantities of oils that are non-food grade — often contaminated with pesticide residues — and used for making cheap cosmetics. Rendered oils should also be avoided. These are the waste oils collected from restaurants and then further refined. Refined oils are often sold as "pure," which is legally permissible and sounds promising, but such oils are not good for mixing with essential oils.

THERAPEUTIC INDICATIONS

All vegetable oils can either be taken internally or used externally. Vegetable oils are normally consumed on their own, to obtain the benefits of a particular oil, without the addition of an essential oil. However, taking olive oil for constipation may be complemented by the external application to the abdomen of black pepper (*Piper nigrum*) or ginger oil (*Zingiber officinale*) at a 3 percent dilution in olive oil.

INTERNAL ACTIVITY

Fats or oils are essential to living matter. The beneficial effects to health from ingesting certain vegetable oils cover a wide spectrum. Evening primrose oil, for instance, has produced some remarkable improvements in cases of eczema, while other vegetable oils are used for their vitamin content. Vegetable oils can be taken by adding them to a salad dressing or swallowed straight from a teaspoon. It is best not to include them in cooking because they are changed by heat, thereby reducing or even removing their beneficial properties.

EXTERNAL ACTIVITY

This is limited to the effect the vegetable oil has on skin cells and tissue since vegetable oils, consisting of larger molecules than essential oils, do not penetrate the skin. Vegetable oils can be used to treat a number of skin complaints and the most effective vegetable oil should be chosen for each treatment. For example, evening primrose oil is also indicated for the external treatment of eczema. Suitable vegetable oils can help in the treatment of varicose veins, bruising, inflamed joints, dry and sensitive skin, allergic conditions and reduction of scarring.

COMBINING VEGETABLE OILS WITH ESSENTIAL OILS FOR EXTERNAL USE

Since some vegetable oils are more specialized than others (rose hip, for instance) and are often the heavier ones (like avocado), it is best to make up your essential oil mix using only 20 percent of such an oil. You can then add a lighter, less specific and less expensive vegetable oil to complete the mix.

The severity and type of condition you are treating will also determine the choice and proportions of vegetable and essential oils in the blend. For example, an appropriate blend for a viral condition that causes acne would be 20 percent hazelnut oil for the oily skin, 77 percent sunflower oil and 3 percent essential oils of tea tree (*Melaleuca alternifolia*) and lavender (*Lavandula angustifolia*) for their antiviral and soothing properties. Any essential oil will mix with any vegetable oil; the secret is to combine oils that enhance and complement one another's therapeutic action.

THE PROPERTIES AND EFFECTS OF VEGETABLE OILS USED IN AROMATOLOGY

Name	Characteristics
almond, sweet (*Prunus amygdalus dulcis*)	mild, fairly viscous massage oil; keeps quite well because of its small amount of vitamin E; can calm irritation caused by eczema
apricot kernel (*Prunus armeniaca*)	light textured, easily absorbed; good general-purpose massage oil
avocado (*Persea americana*)	rich, green oil obtained from fruit pulp, viscous and emollient; good for dry and wrinkled skin, thought to penetrate even the lower layers of the skin
evening primrose (*Oenothera biennis*)	contains essential fatty acids, such as gamma linoleic acid (GLA), that the body cannot make itself; taken internally, it helps combat arthritis, eczema, high blood pressure, high cholesterol and PMS — high doses are needed to achieve lasting results, e.g. 4 g a day
hazelnut (*Corylus avellana*)	astringent; useful for oily skin or acne
macadamia (*Macadamia integrifolia*)	silky textured; rich and nutritive for mature and sunburned skins; taken internally, it is said to be a laxative
olive (*Olea europaea*)	viscous and emollient; soothing for inflamed skin, and good for treating bruises and sprains; taken internally, it relieves constipation, and helps prevent high cholesterol and heart disease

THE PROPERTIES AND EFFECTS OF VEGETABLE OILS USED IN AROMATOLOGY	
Name	Characteristics
peach kernel (*Prunus persica*)	contains vitamin A; prevents dehydration
rose hip (*Rosa canina*)	effective on aging skin and eczema, burns, scars and wounds
safflower (*Carthamus tinctorius*)	not one of the more stable oils, so it can turn rancid easily; useful for the external treatment of bruises, inflamed joints, and sprains; taken internally, it is beneficial for bronchial asthma
sesame (*Sesamum indicum*)	fairly stable; good for dry skin and as a sun filter
sunflower (*Helianthus annuus*)	light, not too greasy; good for treating skin diseases and damage like bruising and ulcers; taken internally, it is good for treating bronchial asthma
tamanu (*Calophyllum inophyllum*)	analgesic, anti-inflammatory, healing
wheatgerm (*Triticum vulgare*)	high vitamin E content; useful for adding to other oils to increase their stability; heavy but good for treating dry skin; taken internally, it can help with eczema, indigestion, varicose veins and breaking down cholesterol deposits. *Note:* people with protein/wheat allergy should be cautious and test a small amount first

MACERATED OR INFUSED OILS

WHAT ARE MACERATED OILS?

Macerated oils are obtained by infusing or *macerating* an herb in a vegetable oil. The herb is chopped up and put into a vat of either almond, sunflower or safflower oil, agitated from time to time and left for a few days in the vat (sealed from the air) at room temperature.

For those plants that do not easily yield their essential oils in steam distillation, this is a way of obtaining aromatics along with other fat-soluble molecules that are also therapeutically beneficial.

ORIGINS   The traditional use of herbal oils obtained by maceration dates back to the ancient Egyptians and Greeks, with their unguents, salves, ointments and balms. These are basically all herbal oils since they contain the fat-soluble matter, including the aromatic extracts, of plant material. Their uses are recorded in subsequent pharmacopoeias. By the time of Paracelsus in 1530, there was a switch from maceration to steam distillation.

It is only relatively recently that the practice of combining steam-distilled essential oils with a vegetable carrier oil has established aromatology as separate from herbalism. However, the recognition that some useful essential oils are being excluded from the aromatologist's repertoire, because they are too difficult or costly to distill, has led to a revival in the use of some macerated oils alongside essential oils.

Any medicinal plant can be combined with a vegetable oil in order to obtain an infused or macerated plant oil. Since aromatologists concentrate on the aromatic part of a plant for healing, it is probably most appropriate for them to limit their use of herbal oils to the maceration of aromatic plant material. The herbal oils with no noted essential oil content, like echinacea and devil's claw, are best left to the medical herbalists to prescribe, or for the informed lay person to use for use in first aid and treating minor ailments at home.

At present there are a range of macerated oils available from several mail-order companies and health food stores. It is also possible to make your own (see below).

HOW MACERATED OILS ARE PRODUCED   Maceration of the plant in the virgin, cold-pressed vegetable oil is best conducted over a long period of time. Quality-control checks through technical analysis ensure that all the active ingredients are present and not destroyed in the process; nothing is added or taken away. The solvent action of the vegetable oil draws all the fat-soluble molecules (including essential oils) from the plant. The oil is then filtered before bottling.

You can carry out this process simply at home by half filling an air-tight container with chopped plant material. Add any warmed, cold-pressed vegetable oil with 5 percent wheatgerm oil to increase the storage life. Screw the lid on, set it in a warm place for 2 to 3 weeks and shake from time to time. Strain the contents through a jelly bag or piece of muslin before bottling. The result is a ready-to-use massage oil.

It is wisest to use up macerated oils as quickly as possible. They go rancid within a few months.

THE USE OF MACERATED OILS   The macerated oils most commonly used by aromatologists are probably calendula, lime blossom, meadowsweet, melissa and St. John's wort. The most popular uses have been for treating aches and pains, inflammation and strains. For more details, please refer to the chart below.

QUANTITIES

Aromatologists tend to apply macerated oils externally in a 3 to 10 percent blend with a vegetable oil. A small amount of essential oil may also be added to complement the mix.

THE PROPERTIES AND EFFECTS OF MACERATED OILS USED IN AROMATOLOGY	
Name	Characteristics
arnica (*Arnica montana*)	used to treat bruising and sprains, chilblains and rheumatic pains; some people can be sensitive to frequent use
calendula (*Calendula officinalis*)	anti-inflammatory and wound healing; good for treating dry eczema, cracked skin and nipples; helps heal skin eruptions and sores, burns and rashes
lime blossom (*Tilia europaea*)	soothing to the skin; aids digestion and sleep
meadowsweet (*Spiraea ulmaria*)	sedative; useful for localized pain relief, e.g. sprains and stiff joints
melissa (*Melissa officinalis*)	useful for treating mature skin and water retention in the legs
mullein (*Verbascum thapsus*)	antiseptic; soothing for neuralgia and rheumatic inflammation; recommended for treating chilblains, hemorrhoids and wounds
St. John's wort (*Hypericum perforatum*)	for treating hard, bruised skin, ulcers and varicose veins; like an embrocation, it increases blood supply to the injured area; rubbed in or applied in a compress, it can relieve the pain of gout, lumbago and rheumatic inflammation in joints

9

BUYING AND STORING ESSENTIAL OILS

To heal with essential oils you must use the natural, distilled or expressed plant extract. You need to know that careful attention has been given to monitoring the plant during all its stages — from growth through harvesting, distillation or expression, and storage.

QUALITY CONTROL

In order to be sure of producing good-quality oils, it is crucial to start out with the highest-quality plant material. This will be determined by such factors as methods of cultivation, soil conditions, seasonal variations, positioning, country of origin and the harvesting time and technique.

Since steam distillation, and to a lesser extent cold pressing or expression, can alter the quality of the original plant material, it is also important to have confidence in the methods used. The control of pressure used in expression or of heat in steam distillation, along with the length of time taken, should be considered. Generally speaking, the lower the pressure and the longer the distillation, the better the end product will be. The use of stainless-steel equipment, spring water and fresh, rather than dried, plant material at the site of picking are all preferable.

I witnessed a quaint example of how *not* to distill an essential oil when I was at a hill station in southern India. I followed my nose to a home distillery: the air was saturated with eucalyptus as decongesting and as penetrating as an inhalation. A hut made of eucalyptus leaves and branches was almost hidden under dense piles of more dried and curled gum foliage. It crackled underfoot as I waded my way through to the entrance.

Inside, a fire pit had been dug into the mud floor, and blue smoke twirled through a hole in the leaf roof. Over the smoldering fire was a rusted, metal drum. Eucalyptus oil was dripping into a chipped tin mug out of a kinked pipe coming from the drum.

I was welcomed by a man and his son who ran the operation together. They gave me the mug of oil to smell. It nearly blew my head off! I would not want to hazard a guess at how many times the foliage was recycled. The local cooperative collects and sells the oil on the open market. It was offered to me as suitable for medical purposes!

Are Oils Derived from Organically Grown Plants Best?

Oils described as *organic* mean that the plants they come from have been grown to certified organic standards. The process, involving tests and inspections, is expensive and the costs are reflected in the higher price asked for these oils.

Just as organically grown fruit and vegetables have more flavor, organic oils can have more "body." Although it is desirable to grow plants naturally, without the use of fertilizers and pesticides, it is impossible to keep crops completely free of the atmospheric pollution we suffer today. Acid rain, radioactive and radium contamination are harder to control than the use of pesticides. These factors have to be considered when weighing up the merits of using organic oils against the extra costs involved in producing them.

It is obviously more natural for a plant to take the nitrogen, phosphate and potassium (known as NPK) it requires from the soil rather than be given the chemically produced NPK. Interestingly, the NPK molecules, whether organically derived or chemically produced, are in either case too large to come through the distillation process. What is more, "organic" is not always synonymous with "good quality." Badly distilled or poor-grade plants, whether organically grown or not, will yield an inferior oil.

On the whole, I would be content to buy from producers and suppliers who sought to work as naturally as possible with plants to produce "whole" oils as close as possible in their composition to the way nature intended them to be.

COPIES

Chemical copies or reconstituted oils may make you feel better because they smell nice, but they can neither reproduce all the chemical properties, in their varying proportions, of the natural plant oil, nor replicate the therapeutic effects.

These synthetic or "nature-identical" oils are all sold under the label of "essential" oils and can confuse the inexperienced buyer. It is only quite recently that a small but growing demand for natural, unadulterated essential oils has come about in response to the increase in their medicinal use. The market is, however, still dominated by the food and flavorings industries, where the need for uniformity is greater than the need for authenticity.

GRADING ESSENTIAL OILS

Frequently essential oils are rectified or adjusted to a common standard by adding or deleting certain chemical constituents, making them conform to the quantities present in a previous batch. The oils are then grouped as Commercial, Pharmaceutical, Industrial, Natural, etc., each with its own grade. For example, lower-grade, "Commercial" ylang ylang is intended for the bottom end of the toiletry market. The problem is that someone could be tempted by the lower price and misled into buying such an oil for therapeutic purposes.

There are also unscrupulous dealers who dilute or alter essential oils and sell them to unsuspecting people for use in aromatherapy. They might dilute an essential oil with a vegetable carrier oil, or remove a cheaper component from one oil and add it or a synthetic one to a more expensive oil to make up the quantity. These are still sold as pure essential oils!

It is easy to recognize an essential oil that has been mixed with a vegetable carrier because it will leave a greasy mark on blotting paper. However, it is difficult to tell whether more camphor or some other ingredient has been used to make up an oil unless you have a very educated nose. With time and practice in smelling different oils you can begin to discern the fakes because they often smell artificial — too pungently of the raw material.

WHERE TO BUY

It is best to buy essential oils for therapeutic use from a recognized health care supplier such as a health food store or mail-order company specializing in this area (as listed under "Helpful Addresses").

It is advisable to steer clear of the outlets that mix health and beauty care products because it is often difficult to tell whether the products have been selected for medicinal or cosmetic use in mind. I know of retailers who claim their brand of toiletry can help clear dandruff or acne but the oils contained in the products are reconstituted ones used by the company's perfume department.

Essential oils sold in transparent glass bottles with no verifiable product information but a tempting price are best resisted. I have had countless clients report skin irritations or nausea as a result of using such products.

WHAT TO BUY

The following is a list of points to consider when you are purchasing pure, natural, distilled or expressed plant oils.

- Dark-glass bottles with integral droppers and screw tops are a good starting point.

- Botanical names are important when selecting the oil you want to buy. They will accurately define the species and even the variety of plant from which the oil originates. The common name may be given but they can be confusing especially in the case of lavender, rosemary, marjoram and chamomile. You should be guided by the Latin name in order to know exactly what you are getting.

- The key chemical constituents should be given for each oil in order to allow you to determine its likely characteristics. At the very least, the listing of these components can make you more aware of how one species of lavender is different from another.

- Cautionary labels are used by some companies who wish to flag certain oils as hazardous. It should be remembered that all oils should be treated with care and what is thought hazardous in one country may be deemed safe in another.

- Sell-by dates are not normally marked on bottles of essential oils. Without these, or at least a bottling date, it is impossible to know how long an oil has been kept in a producer's or supplier's stocks. Try to buy from companies that guarantee they only sell oils produced from the current year's harvest.

- The price should reflect the current availability and demand. Essential oils differ widely in price because the yield varies from plant to plant and from harvest to harvest.

- The aroma of an oil should be dynamic, with depth and vigor. It should not smell too artificially of the plant from which it originates. Not all essential oils smell pleasant.

STORAGE

You should buy essential oils in dark-glass bottles because they deteriorate in sunlight. Deterioration happens faster at the blue end of the spectrum than the red, so black or brown glass is better than blue. It is also advisable to store these bottles in a dark cupboard away from direct sunlight.

Essential oils are volatile so a screw top should always be securely tightened. If the bottle were left open, the oil would eventually evaporate or enough of the lighter molecules would be released and leave an oil with a different composition.

Essential oils are powerful and concentrated substances not to be used in large quantities. Integral droppers inserted in all bottles containing essential oils will help prevent overuse. They also limit spillage, which is useful because the chemicals in the oils can damage plastic, painted or varnished surfaces.

A warm place such as over a radiator is not suitable for storing an essential oil. If the bottle is partly used, the oxygen in the air space can react with the remaining oil.

Oils that are stored in filled and airtight amber bottles in a dark, cool place will keep the longest. Although there are reports of oils lasting for years, it is safest to count on a life of two years for essential oils if kept in these optimum conditions.

Oils with a high aldehyde content, such as those in the citrus group, do not have as long a life. The aldehydes quickly turn to acids so that the oil takes on an acidic smell.

When essential oils are mixed with a lotion, cream or vegetable oil, their shelf life is only as long as that of the product they have been mixed with. For example, a vegetable oil with no preservatives will go rancid after about six months.

10

ESSENTIAL OILS IN HEALTH CARE SETTINGS

ALL IN A MASSAGE?

Many people assume that an aromatherapy treatment means a massage using essential oils. I prefer to call this an *aromatic massage*. Massage is a discipline in its own right to which fragrances may be added to heighten the sensuous and relaxing experience.

In India, where I observed many ayurvedic treatments, I discovered that massage could mean an application of any form of herbal oil to the skin. Dermal penetration of the ayurvedic preparations, which include some essential oils, is carried out by using hot rice poultices containing oils or by a vigorous rubdown with ladles of warm vegetable oil containing herbs and aromatics. The benefits obtained by absorbing the herbs are of primary importance, while the massage itself is only a vehicle with little value attached to what it may contribute in its own right.

MASSAGE IN AROMATOLOGY

The Frenchman René-Maurice Gattefossé, who coined the term *aromatherapy*, did not envisage the use of or necessarily include massage in his work. *Aromatology*, together with *phytotherapy* (herbal medicine), is practiced in France today by medical doctors with a specialty in complementary medicine; it is considered a branch of medicine. The use of essential oils is favored for fighting infections, especially those of the respiratory tract. The methods of application include inhalations, compresses, internal dosage — either oral or through suppositories and pessaries — baths and a limited amount of massage.

MASSAGE IN AROMATHERAPY

In the U.S., Canada, Australia, Great Britain, the Republic of Ireland, South Africa, Israel and some European countries essential oils are mainly used to restore and maintain mental, physical and emotional health by trained nonmedical practitioners or interested medical staff, such as nurses or midwives. These people commonly refer to themselves as *aromatherapists* and use massage as their main way of healing with essential oils.

Training standards, the degree of medical knowledge and scientific understanding of essential oils vary between and within these countries. Although the practice of aromatherapy in these contexts has been growing since the late 1980s, it is in varying stages of infancy in most English-speaking countries.

In the early days — the 1960s onward — and even in some countries today, a rather superficial training in the theory of essential oils went hand in glove with a qualification in massage. Even when I started in the mid-1980s, evidence of my diploma in physiology, anatomy and remedial massage was a prerequisite to my study of and future work with essential oils. Doubtless this heavy bias toward massage as the dominant method of applying essential oils is a result of the cosmetic use beauticians made of oils in facials and body massage in their salons.

Massage and essential oils certainly formed a convenient partnership because essential oils are soluble in the fatty vegetable oil that is used to give the slippage necessary for massage. It was soon found that when blended and applied this way, the fat-soluble essential oils penetrated the skin and entered the blood stream quickly and efficiently. Another reason for the match is that most illness is bound up with experiencing pain and stress. Massage reduces both of these states, while painkilling and sedative oils provide additional relief.

Massage has had the advantage of opening the door in some hospitals and various clinics to the use of essential oils. In some hospitals, for example, doctors were willing to consider the benefits of massage for their patients and tolerated the introduction of essential oils by nurse massage therapists. That the oils might do some good was initially not even considered.

INCREASING ACCEPTANCE OF ESSENTIAL OILS BY TRADITIONAL MEDICAL PRACTITIONERS

More recently, as the therapeutic value of essential oils has gained scientific recognition, there has been an increase in the number of other health professionals and others interested in learning about healing with essential oils. They do not always want to train in massage, and this is supported by the rising number of clients who do not primarily seek a massage. Many more now consult me about specific medical conditions, wanting to be advised on what oils to take and how to apply them at home.

Unfortunately most private health insurance does not pay for complementary therapies but there is a growing acceptance of the part complementary medicine can play in people's health. However, this is a far cry from the use doctors make of essential oils in France, where there is a plethora of pharmacies and analytical laboratories involved in aromatology. A French doctor will have essential oils tested against a sample of bacteria or fungi taken from a patient and order a prescription to be made according to the results of these *aromatograms*.

Worldwide, steps are being taken to broaden the clinical use of essential oils. This trend has encouraged the move away from the term *aromatherapy* toward a new name that reflects *healing* rather than simply *massaging* with essential oils. *Aromatology* embodies this new direction. It neatly avoids the complications implied by the word *therapy* for the Europeans, and the confusion with *aromatic massage* for everyone else.

11

PROFESSIONAL TREATMENT WITH ESSENTIAL OILS

Who Benefits from Treatment?

Anyone can benefit from using essential oils. You have a choice between seeking a consultation for guidance about the selection of essential oils to suit your present condition and methods of home application, or having them applied in massage.

I am commonly asked to help with sinusitis, pre- and postnatal care, eczema, asthma, depression, anxiety, insomnia, muscular strain and pain, fungal and viral infections, PMS, arthritis, ME and irritable bowel syndrome. I prescribe the oils and the best method of application.

I am also asked to give aromatic massage to people who are in need of relaxation and pampering. In this case I am using my skills as a masseuse and choosing a safe oil with a smell that is pleasing to the client rather than drawing on my knowledge as an aromatologist.

WHAT HAPPENS IN A TYPICAL TREATMENT?

The aromatologist will begin with a consultation lasting from between thirty minutes to one hour, depending on the complexity of the case. You will be asked questions about your medical history, general health and lifestyle.

The practitioner should understand the structural make-up, function and diseases of the body, and may wish to contact your physician or any other therapist you are seeing, with your permission, in order to keep all parties informed about any ongoing treatment.

An aromatologist is unlikely to merely focus on the symptoms of illness or imbalance; the underlying causes will be addressed. This may result in recommendations on changes in lifestyle, diet and exercise. For example, in the case of gallstones an attempt may be made to dissolve the stones using oils, or the patient may opt for surgery. In either event the aromatologist will also advise dietary management and the application of essential oils to help the body's conversion of fats or formation of bile.

Many aromatologists may also have training in other disciplines such as nutrition, herbalism or acupuncture, all of which may help in the treatment of particular conditions.

The holistic approach of most complementary medical practitioners means that they will piece together symptoms like a jigsaw puzzle until they get a whole picture of the person seeking treatment. Traditional western medicine attributes illness to exposure to a pathological organism (germ) or to some isolated malfunction in an otherwise healthy body. It then gears its treatment to the specified offender or faulty part.

The aromatologist, on the other hand, steers a middle course, seeing the client as a dynamic whole and the disease as the result of a breakdown in health. Therefore, as well as homing in on the disease itself (such as the application of a bactericidal oil to combat repeated gastroenteritis), the chosen oil would also be a stimulant to the immune system or a tonic to the liver, the kidney or whichever organ is considered to be weakening.

After selecting and blending appropriate oils, the aromatologist suggests the best method of application. This may be through a massage to a part of or the whole body on one or more occasion. It may also be agreed that the client should use the oils at home in compresses or inhalations.

Sessions usually last an hour. If massage or any other application with essential oils is to be given, it may happen at the same time or during a separate visit.

After a massage with oils, most people immediately experience a greater sense of well-being or feel relief from pain or discomfort. I notice that within ten minutes the oils begin to be absorbed and the person visibly relaxes as they take effect.

In some rare cases it is possible to feel very fatigued or develop a headache after a session. This happens when people are debilitated, rundown or full of toxins. The treatment can release toxins from the tissues and produce such reactions as headaches or diarrhea. In addition, the oils can slow down a person who is fighting exhaustion but unable to let go. The solution is to pitch the treatment to a tolerable but effective level, and to administer a series of treatments at four-day intervals.

An aromatologist may follow with advice to exercise, give up smoking or exclude aggravating foods. Attending future appointments and using essential oils in lotions, inhalations or baths at home are suggestions which the practitioner can make but only the client can decide whether to carry out.

It is the practitioner's responsibility to refer the client elsewhere if it is felt that she or he is not skilled or specialized enough to achieve the best results.

How to Find a Qualified Aromatologist

An excellent way to find an aromatologist is by word of mouth. But most countries have a representative body, such as the American Alliance of Aromatherapy. By contacting them (the address is listed under "Helpful Addresses" you can obtain a list of its member associations and training establishments.

Most governing bodies are composed of both aromatherapy associations and training schools. They therefore both unify the profession and establish common standards of training and professional conduct. In addition, they act as a public watchdog and support research in the field.

Questions to Ask

You may find that not all professionals are using the title *aromatologist*, so it would be as well to clarify whether the practitioner uses methods other than massage and what exams he or she has taken in the medical sciences, other complementary therapies and in the theory (including biochemistry) of essential oils.

Ask what length of training a practitioner has undergone. Weekend courses or adult education classes designed to guide people in the use of essential oils at home within the family have been considered sufficient by some to set themselves up as practitioners. Completion of a two-year, part-time course indicates a good level of training, together with the acquisition of other skills in traditional or complementary medicine.

A good practitioner will welcome the following key questions:

- How long did you train?
- To what professional body do you belong?
- What examinations have you taken and passed?

- Are you insured?

- Are you qualified to practice any other therapies?

I am always amazed by the number of people who come to my practice and do not ask any of these questions.

12

CASE STUDIES

The case studies in this chapter are all genuine, although the names have been changed.

CASE ONE: SYLVIA

BACKGROUND

Sylvia's son telephoned me to ask whether I would see his seventy-year-old mother, whom he was very worried about because she had not slept for several days. Her doctor had retired from the local practice. He had been prescribing a sleeping tablet but, after his departure, the tablets had suddenly stopped working.

When Sylvia came to see me the next day, she was very jumpy and overexhausted from lack of sleep. She described herself as generally anxious and fearful of illness striking herself or others. Five days previously she had received some worrying news about a friend's health, which coincided with her own doctor leaving. She took two sleeping tablets that night, followed by another two some hours later. They had no effect. Trying a second night, swallowing the pill to no avail, she decided to give them up altogether. The three following nights, in which she took no sleeping tablets, still brought no sleep.

TREATMENT

Her new doctor had prescribed an antidepressant, which she had taken the previous night. I explained that it was unlikely that these tablets would take immediate effect and remained nonjudgmental about this course of action. At this stage I felt the most important task was to reduce her anxiety and allay her fears about the consequences of her insomnia.

Upon further questioning and physical examination I found that she was in remarkably good health. I advised against taking either caffeine or alcohol in the evenings and recommended an herbal tea containing valerian and chamomile. I finished with a 20-minute back massage using *Lavandula angustifolia* (lavender) and *Ocimum basilicum* (European basil).

In many hospital wards lavender oil has been used in diffusers very successfully in place of medication to induce sleep. I chose the basil because it is helpful with nervous insomnia and debility. It is also indicated for muscle cramps and gastric spasms, both of which were bothering Sylvia.

OUTCOME

Over the next two weeks I repeated this massage treatment four times, taking an hour for each session. Sylvia slowly began to relax and reported an average of five hours' sleep each night. She was experiencing lightheadedness, palpitations and drowsiness during the day because of the antidepressants. With her doctor's knowledge, she decided to reduce the dose gradually with a view to stopping them altogether.

Over the next few weeks there was a steady improvement in Sylvia's sleep pattern. I reduced the treatment sessions but gave Sylvia a bottle of *Lavandula angustifolia* to use in a bath before going to bed and to add to a diffuser in her bedroom. She is now sleeping about six hours a night and is no longer dependent on sleeping tablets.

(See Chapter Three for the discussion about deciding whether to consult a traditional or complementary medical practitioner.)

Case Two: James

Background

A local physiotherapist referred James to me to see whether I could help with the onset of arthritis associated with the Crohn's disease he had had for the last two years. James was twenty-eight years old and was just regaining his strength following a colostomy performed two months ago, in which most of his bowel had been removed.

I found that he was weak, with a lot of inflammation in his lower limbs, and had severe back pain. I decided on the oils I wanted to use but knew that the poor mineral and vitamin absorption that accompanies Crohn's disease, together with the strong medication used, would make James hypersensitive.

I have noticed that anyone convalescing from a serious illness involving heavy medication and/or a breakdown in their immune defense system, such as in the case of HIV-positive patients, is likely to be intolerant to many substances, including essential oils. These therefore must be diluted and mixed with care.

Treatment

I took a skin patch test for *Achillea millefolium* (yarrow) and found that James developed an itchy rash almost immediately. I then tried *Matricaria chamomilla* (German chamomile) and other oils from the Compositae family — the family to which both yarrow and chamomile belong. It was clear from the negative reaction that I was only going to be able to use these oils at a 1 percent dilution in sunflower oil.

Mentha x piperita (peppermint) is another possible skin irritant, but I wanted to use it for its anti-inflammatory effect. James unfortunately complained of an itching sensation after using a very small amount in a back massage. I rubbed generous quantities of a plain vegetable oil over the irritated area then wiped away the excess to relieve the sensation. There was neither a rash nor redness but I decided to find an alternative oil.

I chose *Cinnamomum zeylanicum* (cinnamon bark), which has a high content of cinnamic aldehyde — aldehydes are a good anti-inflammatory but are known to be potential skin sensitizers. However, by carefully blending this oil with *Citrus sinensis* (sweet orange), I was able to "quench" the aldehyde with the large amount of terpene present in the orange oil. Sweet orange is also a useful digestive.

OUTCOME

In each weekly twenty-minute session, by alternating and combining several oils while limiting the overall use of these oils, I achieved good results. Through this careful management and blending of oils, beneficial treatment proceeded without causing any unpleasant or uncomfortable reactions.

(See Chapter Four for information about intolerant reactions to certain essential oils.)

CASE THREE: SUSIE

BACKGROUND

Susie, a twenty-two-year-old receptionist, came to see me about her eczema, which had developed during puberty. Odd patches had appeared on her legs and arms as a child but now large areas of her back, her hands, her knee and elbow joints and her face were affected. She had stopped oral contraception two months ago and experienced a flare-up ever since.

Her periods had been irregular before taking the Pill and she hadn't had one at all since stopping. She complained that she felt she looked very old and that she even felt stiff, which she found disturbing given her age.

I explained that the continual use of cortisone cream inevitably ages and thins the skin. I suspected that the reaction to stopping the Pill would be particularly severe until hormonal activity settled down again.

TREATMENT

I made a cream containing 10 percent evening primrose oil, 2 percent *Matricaria chamomilla* (German chamomile) and 2 percent *Lavandula angustifolia* (lavender) for her to use at home.

I also advised the exclusion of all wheat, dairy and alcoholic products from her diet. This meant Susie would have to devise meal plans because she was used to picking up take-out food and sweet snacks. In addition, she agreed to drink as much water as she could in a day.

I advised that she take two 1000 mg capsules of evening primrose oil morning and evening, and one teaspoon of macadamia nut oil a day (for constipation).

Susie came for weekly treatments in which I used cool compresses of *Hyssopus officinalis* (hyssop), *Juniperus communis* (juniper berry) and *Salvia sclarea* (clary sage) on the affected areas of skin.

After four sessions her skin was less inflamed and some areas had cleared enough to start massage treatment with a 5 percent dilution of evening primrose oil and 5 percent rose hip oil in almond oil containing *Mentha x piperita* (peppermint) and *Hyssopus officinalis*. Although large quantities of peppermint oil can irritate the skin, small amounts can relieve the itching and inflammation that accompanies eczema.

OUTCOME

Within six weeks Susie had her first period since stopping the Pill. We then timed our sessions to fall once a month before her period was due. Over the next six months her periods became regular, her skin was clear other than when she had a dietary lapse and it quickly resolved itself if she applied the cream. Both the constipation and the stiffness disappeared with the course of massage treatment and dietary changes.

CASE FOUR: PETER

BACKGROUND

Peter had suffered from acne on his upper back and face since he was sixteen years old. He was now twenty and in the middle of a course of Roacutain, an oral treatment for acne based on vitamin A. The acne had cleared but the side effects of chapped lips and very dry skin were making him uncomfortable. He was concerned that I would use an oil that would encourage his skin to become oily again, but he did want to have something to relieve the taut, dry cracking.

TREATMENT

I mixed a 3 percent dilution of *Melaleuca alternifolia* (tea tree) with hazelnut oil and gave it to Peter to add to his bath or apply directly, whichever method he felt most comfortable with.

OUTCOME

Peter continued with this treatment for six months since his skin was very dry, but over this period it improved greatly.

Whenever his acne returns and he has to take another course of Roacutain, he comes back to me to replenish his supply of oils.

(For cases Three and Four, see Chapter Eight for information about combining vegetable oils with essential oils.)

CASE FIVE: CHARLES

BACKGROUND

Charles was fifty-five years old when he came to see me about his red and inflamed face; the skin was often chapped and flaking. He knew he could not tolerate something in the atmosphere or in his diet, but he had never isolated what it might be. Although he had a desk-bound job as a civil servant, he spent all his free time either walking or gardening. Apart from prominent varicose veins and the fact that he bruised very easily, he had no other health complaints, except for a permanent feeling of congestion in his sinuses.

Charles felt he did not want to undergo any more tests or trials to identify the allergen or whatever caused his sensitivity. He had a very healthy diet containing no dairy products because he had discovered they increased the congestion in his sinuses. He wondered whether I could alleviate his condition.

TREATMENT

I mixed 2 percent calendula and 2 percent St. John's wort into a cream base containing *Lavandula officinalis* (lavender) for Charles to apply to his face and to his legs. I also gave him a 10 ml bottle of essential oils made up of *Mentha x piperita* (peppermint) and *Eucalyptus radiata* (eucalyptus) in equal proportions. He was to take 6 drops in a steam inhalation every morning.

I recommended that he take 1000 mg of vitamin C morning and evening and increase this dosage and the number of daily inhalations at the first sign of a cold.

OUTCOME

Charles appears for check-up appointments and repeat prescriptions. His face is rarely red now, the skin on his legs is no longer hard and bruised and there are no new varicose veins.

CASE SIX: LIZ

BACKGROUND

Liz, a thirty-four-year-old woman I was helping through her first pregnancy, fell downstairs when she was twenty-nine weeks pregnant. She cracked one rib and was covered in bruises.

TREATMENT

After hospital treatment, I gave Liz pure arnica oil for her partner to massage gently around her rib area. In addition, I advised soaking in baths containing 6 drops of *Lavandula officinalis* (lavender) twice a day.

OUTCOME

After one week of the massage treatment, the pain in Liz's cracked rib had lessened and the bruising and stiffness were considerably reduced.

CASE SEVEN: HELEN

BACKGROUND

Helen, a sixty-year-old woman who ran a boarding kennel for dogs, was finding that when she got up in the morning she could hardly move her fingers and wrists because they had stiffened in the night.

TREATMENT

I mixed 2 percent St. John's wort with 2 percent meadowsweet in a gel containing 3 percent *Zingiber officinale* (ginger) and 1 percent *Piper nigrum* (black pepper). I explained that I had calculated the preparation as well as I could with only these few personal details to guide me, and explained that she should apply the gel to her hands morning and night.

OUTCOME

After one month she ordered another jar and said her hands were pain free and had regained full mobility in the finger joints.

(For cases Five, Six and Seven, see Chapter Eight for information about combining macerated oils with essential oils.)

CASE EIGHT: JANET

BACKGROUND

When Janet, aged thirty-six, came to me she had just finished her fifth course of antibiotics taken within the last twelve months for a chronic urinary tract infection. For the past five years she had suffered from persistent urethritis, involving an urgent and frequent desire to empty the bladder, accompanied by general inflammation and discomfort in the vagina. Janet had stopped taking oral contraception six months ago and wanted to try to get pregnant but sexual intercourse with her partner was too painful.

A recent urine sample taken following the last antibiotic treatment was sent for microbiological investigation and proved to be "sterile." In other words, it did not contain the level of pathogenic bacteria per milliliter of urine required by traditional medicine to confirm a urinary tract infection. Yet Janet was in perpetual misery from her symptoms.

TREATMENT

I sent a vaginal swab and urine samples to a laboratory for microscopy and culture. I then planned my selection of essential oils for treatment according to the findings that the bacteria *Escherichia coli* and *Klebsiella aerogenes* were present in the urino-genital area. The oils known to be active against these bacteria are *Cinnamomum zeylanicum* (cinnamon bark), *Melaleuca leucadendron* (cajuput) and *Thymus vulgaris* ct thymol (red thyme). I then double-checked the validity of my stock of these oils with an aromatogram, and introduced them in turn to the culture grown in the laboratory.

I included *Melaleuca alternifolia* (tea tree) because the long-term use of broad-spectrum antibiotics had also caused a candidiasis infection, popularly known as vaginal thrush, with the yeast-like fungus *Candida albicans*.

These 4 oils were mixed in equal proportions in a 50 percent dilution with sunflower oil and applied 3 times a week in a 15-minute abdominal and lower-back massage. For home use, I mixed a 3 percent dilution of *Zingiber officinale* (ginger) and *Mentha x piperita* (peppermint) in equal proportions in sunflower oil to help with the constipation and the pain and inflammation respectively. This was to be applied to the abdominal area once a day. I advised the nightly insertion of tampons soaked in 10 ml live yogurt containing 10 drops of *Melaleuca alternifolia* to further combat the thrush.

Dietary changes were necessary, too — vital for the successful treatment of thrush. Sugars, fermented foods, alcohol and other aggravants were slowly excluded over the next four weeks. In addition, I recommended a high fluid intake to flush out the bladder and to relieve the constipation. Janet took 6 acidopholus tablets a day in order to replenish the intestinal flora that would have been adversely affected by the courses of antibiotics she had taken.

OUTCOME

By the end of the month there was no vaginal discharge, itching, pain or inflammation. Janet said she felt revitalized and free from the permanent tiredness that had blighted everything. For the following six months the above treatment was repeated for the three days before menstruation because the symptoms would recur to a moderate degree at this time. In September of that year Janet conceived, and she now has a healthy son.

(See Chapter Ten for the discussion about how aromatology can be complementary to traditional medical care.)

CASE NINE: DOMINIC

BACKGROUND

Dominic, a forty-one-year-old financial trader who worked long days at his desk in a bank, sought my help in 1990 because he was feeling generally unwell and fatigued.

I took some preliminary information about his height, weight and previous medical history. He was over six-feet tall and slightly overweight; he enjoyed daily business lunches with alcohol and had a glass of whisky every evening. Although he tried to get to the gym three times a week, his life was otherwise sedentary.

In 1989, following five years of chronic cholecystitis (inflammation of the gall bladder), his gall bladder was removed. He still suffered from intermittent colicky abdominal pain, similar to what he had experienced before the surgery, but diarrhea was a new, additional symptom. He complained of a tight feeling across the site of the operation. Upon examination I found the scar tissue was hard, prominent and irregular and that his abdomen was bloated.

In the last year Dominic had had frequent severe headaches for the first time in his life. He complained of stiffness in his neck and shoulders. He was tall and was often bent over his desk. It turned out, too, that he frequently hooked his telephone between his chin and his shoulder while keying into his computer. I recommended the use of telephone headsets and a course in Alexander technique to make him aware of his posture.

I suspected the headaches and the abdominal discomfort were connected and related to the history of large gallstones, a problem that had been relieved but not solved by the removal of his gall bladder. He had continued with a high-fat, high-protein diet, accompanied by high alcohol consumption. I advised dietary changes to a low-fat, high-fiber diet without caffeine or alcohol. I suggested that we might experiment with the type and amount of fiber he introduced into his meals because symptoms of irritable bowel syndrome can get worse before they adapt and improve with such changes.

TREATMENT

Treatment consisted of massage sessions once a week, using slightly sedative oils to settle the digestive system and relax the muscles. The mixtures of oil were 10 percent dilutions in safflower and rose hip oils of any 4 of the following: *Lavandula angustifolia* (lavender), *Achillea millefolium* (yarrow), *Matricaria chamomilla* (German chamomile), *Citrus limon* (lemon), *Mentha x piperita* (peppermint) and *Citrus aurantium* var. *amara* (per.) (orange Bigarade).

OUTCOME

After six weeks Dominic reported only back pain. He had changed his diet considerably and felt that he had renewed energy. We decided to continue with body massage to relax and loosen his muscles in conjunction with more regular workouts involving stretch exercise and aerobic activity to achieve weight loss and greater mobility.

(See Chapter Eleven for the description of the holistic approach of aromatologists.)

HELPFUL ADDRESSES

AROMATHERAPY ASSOCIATIONS

Aromatherapy associations keep lists of approved training establishments and/or qualified therapists. They also provide a code of practice and guidance on matters arising from treatment and practice.

◆ **American Alliance of Aromatherapy**
PO Box 309
Depoe Bay, OR 97341
Tel.: 503-392-4006 or 800-809-9850
◆ Fax: 503-392-4544 or 800-809-9808

American Botanical Council
PO Box 201660
◆ Austin, TX 78720-1660
Tel.: 512-331-8868
Fax: 512-331-1924

American Herbalist Guild
PO Box 746555
Arvada, CO 80006
Tel.: 303-423-8800
Fax: 303-402-1564

Aromatherapy Institute and Research
PO Box 2354
Fair Oaks, CA 95628
Tel.: 916-965-7546
Fax: 916-962-3292

Herb Research Foundation
1007 Pearl Street, Suite 200
Boulder, CO 80302
Voice mail: 800-748-2617, 303-449-2265

National Association for Holistic Aromatherapy
PO Box 17622
Boulder, CO 80308-7622
Tel.: 415-731-4634
Fax: 415-564-6799

Aromatherapy Training

Many of these training schools have branches or colleges in other countries.

International Federation of Aromatherapists
Stamford House, 2–4 Chiswick High Road,
London W4 1TH
Tel.: 0181 742 2605

International Society of Professional Aromatherapists
Hinckley and District Hospital and Health Centre,
The Annex, Mount Road, Hinckley, Leicestershire LE10 1AG
Tel.: 01455 637987

London School of Aromatherapy
The Swanfleet Centre, 93 Fortress Road,
London NW5 1AG
Tel.: 0171 267 6717

The Raworth Centre
College for Sports Therapy and Natural Medicine,
20–26 South Street, Dorking
Surrey RH4 2HQ
Tel.: 01306 742150

Shirley Price International College of Aromatherapy
Essentia House, Upper Bond Street, Hinckley, Leicestershire LE10 1RS
Tel. 01455 633231

The Tisserand Aromatherapy Institute
65 Church Road, Hove, East Sussex BN3 2BD
Tel.: 01273 206640

Aromatherapy Products

Many companies distribute worldwide. Send a stamped, addressed envelope when you write for price lists.

USA

Aroma Vera Inc.
1830 Robertson Boulevard #203
Los Angeles, CA 90035
Tel.: 310-280-0407

Ledet Aromatic Oils
PO Box 2354
Fair Oaks, CA 95628

United Kingdom

The Aromatherapy Trade Council
PO Box 52, Market Harborough
Leicestershire LE16 8ZX
Tel.: 01858 465731
Send a stamped, addressed envelope for general information and a list of members and recognized suppliers.

The Fragrant Earth Co. Ltd
PO Box 182, Taunton
Somerset TA1 1YR
Tel.: 01823 335734

New Seasons
The Old Post Office, Lockinge, Wantage,
Oxfordshire OX12 8PA
Tel.: 01235 821110

Phoenix Natural Products
15 Witley Industrial Estate, Southall
Middlesex UB2 4EZ
Tel.: 0181 574 7308

Shirley Price Aromatherapy Ltd
Essentia House, Upper Bond Street, Hinckley
Leicestershire LE10 1RS
Tel.: 01455 615466
Fax: 01455 615054

PUBLICATIONS
International Journal of Aromatherapy
PO Box 750428
Petaluma, CA 94975-0428
Tel.: 800-809-9845

RECOMMENDED READING

———

Belaiche, P., *Phytothérapie et aromathérapie*, Paris: Maloine, 1979.

Chaitow, Leon, *Soft Tissue Manipulation*, London: Thorsons, 1988.

Davis, Patricia, *Aromatherapy: An A–Z*, Saffron Walden: C. W. Daniel, 1988.

Franchomme, Pierre and Pénoël, Daniel, *L'Aromathérapie exactement: encyclopédie de l'utilisation thérapeutique des huiles essentielles* (ed. Roger Jollois), Limoges: 1990.

Gattefossé, René-Maurice, *Aromathérapie*, Paris: Girardot 1937; *Gattefossé's Aromatherapy* (English tr.), Saffron Walden: C. W. Daniel, 1993.

Gumbel, Dietrich, *Principles of Holistic Skin Therapy with Herbal Essences* (tr. Ritva Abao), Heidelberg: Karl F. Haug, 1986.

Lautié, Raymond and Passebecq, André, *Aromatherapy: The Use of Plant Sources in Healing*, London: Thorsons, 1979.

Mailhebiau, Philippe, *La Nouvelle Aromathérapie*, Toulouse: Vie Nouvelle, 1989.

Price, Shirley, *The Aromatherapy Workbook*, London: Thorsons, 1993.

Price, Shirley and Len, *Aromatherapy for Health Professionals*,
    Edinburgh: Churchill Livingstone, 1995.

Valnet, Jean, *The Practice of Aromatherapy*, Saffron Walden: C. W.
    Daniel, 1982.

INDEX

Abrasions and cuts, 43, 57
Abscesses, 42
Absolutes, 3–4
Aches and pains, 39, 40, 41, 44, 50, 51
Acids, 23
Acne, 37, 50, 66
Alcohols, 23–24
Aldehydes, 19, 24
Allergic reactions, 20–21
Almond (*Prunus amygdalus dulcis*), 67
Analyzing of essential oils, 5
Angelica (*Angelica archangelica*), 21, 27
Aniseed (*Pimpinella anisum*), 24, 29
Antibiotics, 14
Antigens, 20
Appetite loss, 41
Application methods, 2–3, 41, 49–61
Apricot kernel (*Prunus armeniaca*), 67

Arnica (*Arnica montana*), 71
Aromatherapists, 80
Aromatherapy, 7, 10
  and massage, 80–81
  origin of term, 7, 9
Aromatic massage, 10, 79
Aromatograms, 82
Aromatologists, 11, 84–87
Aromatology, 7, 11, 82
  and massage, 80
Arthritis, 37, 51
Asthma, 36–37, 39, 40, 48, 60
Athlete's foot, 39, 42
Avicenna, 3, 8
Avocado (*Persea americana*), 67

Bad breath, 40
Bath dispersants, 49
Baths, 49–50, 53–54
Bergamot (*Citrus bergamia*), 25, 30
Bites, insect, 36, 40, 44, 51, 52
Black pepper (*Piper nigrum*), 30, 65

Black pepper oil, 2
Bleeding gums, 42, 58
Blue gum (*Eucalyptus globulus*), 36–37
Boils, 36, 42, 51, 52
Botanical families, 27–32
Botany, and essential oils, 27–33
Bottles, 5, 17, 61, 62, 76, 77
    labels, 19–20, 31, 76
Bronchial complaints, 41. *See also* Colds; Coughs; *etc.*
Bronchitis, 36–37
Bruises, 42, 51, 53, 57, 66
Burns and scalds, 38, 42

Cajuput (*Melaleuca leucadendron*), 27
Calendula (*Calendula officinalis*), 71
Caraway (*Carum carvi*), 24, 27, 30, 35
Carbon dioxide extraction, 3
Carriers for essential oils, 47
Case studies, 88–99
Catarrh, 42, 60
Cedarwood (*Cedrus atlantica*), 30
Cellulite, 42
Chamomile. *See* German chamomile
Chemical families, 23–27
Chemical properties of essential oils, 5, 23–27
Chemical variability in essential oils, 26- 27
Chemotypes, 32
Chest infections, 60
Chilblains, 42
Cinnamon bark (*Cinnamomum zeylanicum*), 2, 24, 29
Citrus oils, 2, 3. *See also specific citrus oils*

Clary sage (*Salvia sclarea*), 29
Clay packs, 50
Clove (*Syzygium aromaticum*), 25, 30
Cold pressing, 3, 64
Cold sores, 42
Colds, 36, 40, 42, 43, 48, 51, 52, 60
Colitis, 38
Combinations/blends
    of essential oils, 55–61
    of essential/vegetable oils, 55–56, 66
Complementary care, 12–15, 79–81
Compresses, 51–52
Constipation, 41, 42
Conventional health care, 12–15, 81–82
Coriander (*Coriandrum sativum*), 27, 30
Coughs, 36, 40, 43, 60
Coumarins, 25
Cramps, 39, 43
Creams and massage, 56–57
Cultivars, 32
Cuts and abrasions, 43, 57
Cypress (*Cupressus sempervirens*), 29
Cystitis, 36–37, 38, 43

Dandruff, 43, 59, 60–61
Dental surgery, 58
Depression, 56
Dermatitis, 43
Devil's claw, 69–70
Diabetes, 36–37
Diaper rash, 43
Diffusers, 52
Digestion tonic, 37
Digestive problems. *See* Indigestion; Nausea; *etc.*

Dioscorides, 8
Dosages of essential oils, 17–18, 62
Droppers, 5–6, 17, 76, 77
Dry hair, 59
Dry skin, 50, 57

Echinacea, 69–70
Eczema, 37, 38, 43, 54
Egyptians, ancient, 4, 8, 69
Essential oils
    analyzing, 5
    application methods, 2–3, 41, 46, 49–61
    botany, 27–33
    chemical properties, 5, 23–27
    defined, 2
    dosages, 17–18, 62
    extraction methods, 3–4, 72–73
    grading, 75
    healing methods, 46–62
    history, 1, 7–11
    marketing, 4–5
    price, 77
    purchasing, 5–6, 72–77
    safety, 16–21
    shelf life, 6, 77–78
    sources, 2
    storage, 6, 61, 62, 77–78
Esters, 23
Eucalyptus (Eucalyptus globulus), 25, 30, 36–37
Europe, and herbalism, 8–10
European basil (Ocimum basilicum), 29
Evening primrose (Oenothera biennis), 65, 66, 67
Extraction methods, 3–4, 72–73

Face packs, 50
Fainting, 40

Fatigue, 40, 43
Fennel (Foeniculum vulgare), 30
Fever, 36, 37
Flatulence, 40, 41
Fleas, 43
Fluid retention, 43
Foot baths, 53–54
France, 9–10, 80
Franchomme, Pierre, 10
Frankincense (Boswellia carteri), 29
Furocoumarins, 19, 21, 25

Gargles, 54
Gas-liquid chromatograph, 5, 26
Gastritis, 38
Gattefossé, René-Maurice, 9–10, 80
Gels and massage, 57–58
Genus of plants, 28
Geranium (Pelargonium graveolens), 29
German chamomile (Matricaria chamomilla), 24, 29, 38–39
German measles, 43
Ginger (Zingiber officinale), 2, 30, 41, 65
Gingivitis, 43
Gout, 37
Grading of essential oils, 75
Great Britain, 10, 13
Greeks, ancient, 1, 8, 69
Gums, bleeding, 42, 58

Hair care, 59, 60–61
Hand baths, 53–54
Hangover, 43
Hay fever, 39, 43
Hazelnut (Corylus avellana), 67
Head colds, 48, 51, 52. See also Colds
Head lice, 44, 60–61

Headaches, 38, 40, 44, 48, 51, 52
Healing methods, 46–62
Heartburn, 44
Heat rash/bumps, 44
Hemorrhoids, 44, 59
Herbal extracts, 19
Herbal oils, 69–71
Herbalism, 7, 8, 18–19
Herpes, 39
Hiccups, 44
Hippocrates, 1
History of essential oils, 1,
    7–11
Hot extractions, 64
Hybrids, 32
Hyssop (*Hyssopus officinalis*), 20,
    24, 29

India, 4–5, 8, 73, 79
Indigestion, 38–39, 40, 41, 44
Infections, 35, 39
Inflammation, reducing, 51
Influenza, 44
Inhalation of essential oils, 41,
    48, 53, 60
Insect bites, 36, 40, 44, 51, 52
Insomnia, 38, 44, 52, 53, 56
Internal use of essential oils,
    2–3, 16, 17, 48
Intestinal parasites, 36–37
Intolerance to substance, 21
Irritable bowel syndrome, 40

Jacuzzis, 54
Juniper berry (*Juniperus commu-
    nis*), 29, 37

Ketones, 19, 24

Labels, on bottles, 19–20, 31, 76
Lactones, 25
Laryngitis, 44

Latin names of plants, 28, 31, 76.
    See also specific plants
Lavender (*Lavandula
    angustifolia*), 17, 23, 29, 37–38
Lavender (*Lavandula officinalis*),
    37–38, 47
Lavender (*Lavandula stoechas*),
    31
Lavender (*Lavandula vera*), 23,
    31, 37–38
Leg ulcers, 38
Lemon (*Citrus limon*), 2, 30,
    35–36
Lemongrass (*Cymbopogon citra-
    tus*), 24
Lethargy, 37, 56
Lice, 44, 60–61
Light-bulb ring, 53
Lilac oil, 2
Lime (*Citrus medica* var.
    vulgaris), 30
Lime blossom (*Tilia europaea*),
    71
Liver tonic, 36
Lotions and massage, 56–57

Macadamia (*Macadamia integri-
    folia*), 67
Macerated oils, 69–71
Marigold (*Tagetes minuta*), 29
Marjoram oil, 2
Marketing of essential oils, 4–5
Massage, 2, 47–48, 54–58, 79–81
Maury, Marguerite, 10
Meadowsweet (*Spiraea ulmaria*),
    71
Melissa (*Melissa officinalis*), 71
Memory loss, 40
Menstrual problems, 40
Mineral oil, 54
Mouth ulcers, 44, 58
Mouth washes, 58

Mullein (*Verbascum thapsus*), 71
Muscular aches and pains. *See* Aches and pains
Myrrh (*Commiphora myrrha*), 29
Myrtle (*Myrtus communis*), 2, 27, 30

"Nature-identical" oils, 74
Nausea, 44
Neroli (*Citrus aurantium* var. *amara*), 30
Neuralgia, 45
Niaouli (*Melaleuca viridiflora*), 30

Oils. *See* Essential oils; *see also* specific plant oil or oil type
Oily hair, 59
Oily skin, 50
Olive (*Olea europaea*), 65, 67
Orange (*Citrus aurantium*), 2, 25, 30
Organic oils, 73–74
Oxides, 25

Paracelsus, 9, 69
Patch test, 21
Patchouli (*Pogostemon patchouli*), 6
Peach kernel (*Prunus persica*), 68
Pennyroyal (*Mentha pulegium*), 19
Peppermint (*Mentha x piperita*), 29, 39–40
Percolation, 3
Perfumery, 7, 9–10, 19
Pessaries, 48
Phenols, 19, 25
Photosynthesis, 32
Phytotherapy (herbal medicine), 80
Pine (*Pinus sylvestris*), 30
Plant families, 27–32

Plants, and production of essential oils, 32–33
Pneumonia, 36–37
Post-viral syndrome, 39
Premenstrual syndrome (PMS), 56
Price of essential oils, 77
Purchase of essential oils, 5–6, 72–77

Quinta essentia, 9

Reconstituted oils, 74
Refined oils, 65
Relaxation, 49, 52, 53
Rendered oils, 65
Resinoids, 3–4
Responsibility for own health, 13–14
Revitalization, 49
Rheumatism, 37
Ringworm, 39, 45
Rome, ancient, 8
Room vaporizer, 52–53
Rose hip (*Rosa canina*), 68
Rosemary (*Rosmarinus officinalis*), 29, 40
Rosewood (*Aniba rosaeodora*), 29

Safety with essential oils, 16–21
Safflower (*Carthamus tinctorius*), 68
Sage (*Salvia officinalis*), 20, 24, 29
St. John's wort (*Hypericum perforatum*), 71
Saunas, 59
Scalds. *See* Burns and scalds
Scars and scarring, 38, 66
Sell-by dates, 76–77
Sensitization, 21
Sesame (*Sesamum indicum*), 68
Shampoos, 59

Shelf life of essential oils, 6, 77–78,

Shingles, 45

Shock, 45

Sinusitis, 40, 45, 48, 58, 60

Sitz baths, 59

Skin absorption, 47–48

Skin irritation, and essential oils, 24, 25

Skin problems, 36, 38, 50, 57, 66. *See also specific problems*

Smell of essential oils, 77

Solvent extraction, 3–4

Sore throat and laryngitis, 44, 45, 54

Sources of essential oils, 2

Species of plants, 28

Sprains, 45, 51, 53

Spruce oil, 2

Steam distillation, 3

Steam inhalation, 60

Stiffness and stiff joints, 45, 51, 58. *See also* Aches and pains

Stomach pains, 51

Storage of essential oils, 6, 61, 62, 77–78

Stress and tension, 38, 56

Stretch marks, reducing, 55

Sunburn, 40, 45

Sunflower (*Helianthus annuus*), 61, 68

Sunlight sensitivity, and essential oils, 21, 25

Suppositories, 48

Synthetic oils, 27, 74

Tamanu (*Calophyllum inophyllum*), 68

Taxonomy of plants, 27–32

Tea tree (*Melaleuca alternifolia*), 17, 27, 30, 39, 47

Tension and stress, 38, 56

Terpenes, 25–26

Thrush, 39, 45, 59

Thyme (*Thymus vulgaris*), 29

Thyme (*Thymus vulgaris* ct thujanol-4), 20, 24

Tooth decay, 58

Toothache, 58

Treatment, typical, 84–85

Tuberculosis, 36–37

Urticaria, 38, 45

Vaginal healing after childbirth, 59

Valnet, Jean, 10, 36, 40

Vaporizers, 52–53

Varicose veins, 45, 55, 66

Varieties of plants, 31

Vegetable oils, 49, 54, 61, 63–68 and massage, 54–56

Vertigo, 35, 40

Vetiver (*Vetiveria zizanioides*), 2, 6

Vulvar pruritus, 38

Warts, 36, 45

Wheatgerm (*Triticum vulgare*), 20, 68 as preservative, 61, 70

World War I, and use of essential oils, 10

Yarrow (*Achillea millefolium*), 21

Ylang ylang (*Cananga odorata*), 2, 29

ULYSSES PRESS HEALTH BOOKS

DISCOVER HANDBOOKS

Easy to follow and authoritative, *Discover Handbooks* reveal an array of alternative therapies from around the world and demonstrate how to incorporate them into a program of good health.

Each book opens with information on the history and principles of the particular technique, then presents practical and straightforward guidance on ways in which it can be applied. Offering the tools needed to achieve and maintain an optimal state of health, the approach is one of personal improvement and self-reliance. Each of the books features: an introduction to the discipline; an explanation of its philosophy; step-by-step guide to its implementation; clear diagrams and charts; and case studies.

DISCOVER AYURVEDA
ISBN 1-56975-081-5, 128 pp, $8.95

DISCOVER COLOR THERAPY
ISBN 1-56975-093-9, 144 pp, $8.95

DISCOVER ESSENTIAL OILS
ISBN 1-56975-080-7, 128 pp, $8.95

DISCOVER FLOWER ESSENCES
ISBN 1-56975-099-8, 120 pp, $8.95

DISCOVER MEDITATION
ISBN 1-56975-113-7, 144 pp, $8.95

DISCOVER NUTRITIONAL THERAPY
ISBN 1-56975-135-8, 120 pp, $8.95

DISCOVER OSTEOPATHY
ISBN 1-56975-115-3, 132 pp, $8.95

DISCOVER REFLEXOLOGY
ISBN 1-56975-112-9, 132 pp, $8.95

DISCOVER SHIATSU
ISBN 1-56975-082-3, 128 pp, $8.95

A Natural Approach Books

Written in a friendly, nontechnical style, *A Natural Approach* books address specific health issues and show you how to take an active part in your own treatment. Whether you suffer from panic attacks, endometriosis or depression, each book will provide you with a thorough understanding of your condition and detail organic solutions that offer immediate relief for your symptoms and effectively remedy their underlying causes.

Believing that disease is more than a combination of symptoms, these books offer integrated mind/body programs that take a positive, preventative approach. Since traditional drug therapy is not always the best solution (and can sometimes be the problem), these guides show how to use alternative treatments to supplement or replace conventional medicine.

ANXIETY & DEPRESSION
ISBN 1-56975-118-8, 144 pp, $9.95

IRRITABLE BOWEL SYNDROME
ISBN 1-56975-030-0, 240 pp, $11.95

ENDOMETRIOSIS
ISBN 1-56975-088-2, 120 pp, $8.95

MIGRAINES
ISBN 1-56975-140-4, 156 pp, $8.95

FREE YOURSELF FROM TRANQUILIZERS
& SLEEPING PILLS
ISBN 1-56975-074-2, 192 pp, $9.95

PANIC ATTACKS
ISBN 1-56975-045-9, 148 pp, $8.95

IRRITABLE BLADDER & INCONTINENCE
ISBN 1-56975-089-0, 108 pp, $8.95

The Natural Healer Books

As home remedies and alternative treatments become increasingly accepted into the medical mainstream, people want information—not just hype and unproven claims—about the remedies they see in health food stores. *The Natural Healer* books detail how these natural remedies have been used throughout history and how to safely incorporate them into an overall plan for maintaining good health.

CIDER VINEGAR
ISBN 1-56975-141-2, 120 pp, $8.95

GARLIC
ISBN 1-56975-097-1, 120 pp, $8.95

THE ANCIENT AND
HEALING ARTS BOOKS

The Ancient and Healing Arts books recount the development of healing art forms that have been used for thousands of years. Beautifully illustrated with full color on every page, they discuss the benefits of these time-honored techniques and offer detailed instructions on their use.

THE ANCIENT AND HEALING ART OF
AROMATHERAPY
ISBN 1-56975-094-7, 96 pp, $14.95

THE ANCIENT AND HEALING ART OF
CHINESE HERBALISM
ISBN 1-56975-139-0, 96 pp, $14.95

OTHER HEALTH TITLES

THE BOOK OF KOMBUCHA
ISBN 1-56975-049-1, 160 pp, $11.95
Explains the benefits of and addresses concerns about Kombucha, the widely used Chinese "tea mushroom."

HEPATITIS C: A PERSONAL GUIDE TO GOOD HEALTH
ISBN 1-56975-091-2, 172 pp, $12.95
Identifies the causes and symptoms of hepatitis C and presents conventional and alternative treatments for coping with the disease.

KNOW YOUR BODY: THE ATLAS OF ANATOMY
ISBN 1-56975-021-1, 160 pp, $12.95
Presents a full-color guide to the structure of the human body.

MOOD FOODS
ISBN 1-56975-023-8, 192 pp, $9.95
Shows how the foods you eat influence your emotions and behavior.

YOUR NATURAL PREGNANCY: A GUIDE TO COMPLEMENTARY THERAPIES
ISBN 1-56975-059-9, 240 pp, $16.95
Details alternative therapies ranging from aromatherapy to yoga that can benefit pregnant women.

To order these books call 800-377-2542, fax 510-601-8307 or write to Ulysses Press, P.O. Box 3440, Berkeley, CA 94703-3440. All retail orders are shipped free of charge. California residents must include sales tax. Allow two to three weeks for delivery.

Nicola Naylor is a clinical aromatherapist with private practices in the United Kingdom.